MedSpeak Illuminated

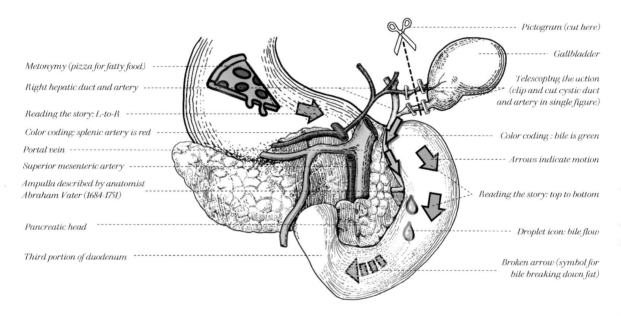

Pictogram (cut here)

Gallbladder

Metonymy (pizza for fatty food)

Right hepatic duct and artery

Telescoping the action
(clip and cut cystic duct
and artery in single figure)

Reading the story: L-to-R

Color coding: splenic artery is red

Color coding : bile is green

Portal vein

Superior mesenteric artery

Arrows indicate motion

Ampulla described by anatomist
Abraham Vater (1684-1751)

Reading the story: top to bottom

Pancreatic head

Droplet icon: bile flow

Third portion of duodenum

Broken arrow (symbol for
bile breaking down fat)

MedSpeak Illuminated

The Art and Practice of Medical Illustration

François I. Luks

The Kent State University Press   Kent, Ohio

To Monique, Valérie, Charlotte, and Sophie:

the best, smartest, most supportive, most—

well, you get the picture . . .

Frontispiece: Biliary function and technique of cholecystectomy (Posterior view of stomach and duodenum). After Henry Vandyke Carter (1918), *Gray's Anatomy*

© 2022 by The Kent State University Press, Kent, Ohio 44242
All rights reserved

Unless otherwise noted, all illustrations are by the author.

ISBN 978-1-60635-443-8
Manufactured in the United States of America

Cataloging information for this title is available at the Library of Congress.

26 25 24 23 22 5 4 3 2 1

Contents

Preface

Ten years ago, I agreed to give a two-hour workshop on medical illustration to first-year medical students. Fortunately, I was not asked to show my credentials in the field of scientific illustration (I have none), but I felt at least somewhat qualified. I have been drawing (and doodling) for most of my childhood and all of my adult life and have accumulated a decent portfolio of medical illustrations—illustrations of my own research work and that of friends and colleagues. I am also a huge medical illustration nerd and have met many extremely talented and experienced medical illustrators along the way, giving me a little bit of street cred by association.

The two-hour workshop struck a nerve, and gradually morphed into a full semester course for undergraduate students at Brown University and the Rhode Island School of Design. To try to make the course interesting (for the students and myself), I interspersed drawing instruction classes with lectures on the history of medical illustration, the parallels between the two professions (doctors and illustrators), the ethical aspects of anatomic dissection and scientific illustration—and I went deeper and deeper down the rabbit hole of medicine in art: the innumerable references to medical conditions and medical practices in classic paintings and sculptures. Most of it had been described plenty of times before, but I stumbled onto a few pearls and undiscovered treasures that I couldn't wait to share with the students. And as I am only an enlightened amateur when it comes to medical illustration, I complemented my own shortcomings with guest appearances by professional illustrators who could fill in the gaps.

The positive reactions of students and colleagues to a course in medical illustration have told me that I am not alone in my fascination with the subject, and many doctor-artists have come out of the proverbial woodwork after finding out about the classes. Many more physicians and academics draw in their daily life (to explain or teach) without calling themselves even budding artists. Clearly, we are all visual communicators, and most of us wouldn't mind getting better at it.

This book is inspired by the course. It is not a syllabus, however, even though parts of it may seem familiar to former students. It is not an authoritative history of medical illustration; it is not a drawing manual; and it is definitely not a scholarly work on art history or the history of medicine. It could be considered fan fiction of any (or all) of the above from the point of view of a weathered academic surgeon with more than a passing interest in medical illustration. I hope that this book will help others appreciate the role of scientific visualization, its place in history, its relevance today, and the lessons it can teach all of us if we want to be better communicators.

Acknowledgments

This project is the result of a virtual meeting brokered by Jay Baruch (skilled emergency medicine physician and brilliant writer), who put me in contact with Susan Wadsworth-Booth, Kent State University Press director and fairy godmother of this book. She was nice enough to listen to me and believed my ideas had potential. Without Jay or Susan, this book would not exist. I am grateful for the friendship and advice of a growing posse of medical illustrators—chief among them Ian Suk, the most gifted artist and nicest person I know; Jill Gregory in New York, Julia Lerner and Vinnie Francis at Brown, Brian Dunham in Philadelphia, and various members of the Association of Medical Illustrators who have been so generous and welcoming. Between the course in medical illustration and our new Medical Comics workshop at Brown, I have relied on many other professionals—Emily Slapin, Deirdre Fearon, Scott Collins, Valerie Weiss, Marguerite Vigliani, Shirlene Obuobi—and they are all present in the book, as is Susan Doyle, chair of the Illustration Department at RISD, and an even greater cheerleader than I am for the possibilities of RISD-Brown partnerships in medical illustration. Thanks also to Julia Wiesenberg, Christine Brooks, Mary Young, and Valerie Ahwee at Kent State University Press for making the final process so smooth. I am ever grateful for the support of Valérie, Charlotte, and Sophie in this and in so many other endeavors. Finally, there is Monique, who came up with the title, is the best (and most brutally honest) proofreader in the world, and whose approval for the final product means everything to me.

Introduction

What Is Medical Illustration?

Medical illustration is a poorly understood profession—not just by the lay public but by many healthcare professionals and scientists as well. If people are a little bit familiar with the term, chances are they will mention Frank Netter, who has taught generations of North American medical professionals. His vivid paintings are appreciated in equal measures for their beautiful, colorful renditions of anatomy, and for a feeling of nostalgia (Fig. 1). Andreas Vesalius will probably be mentioned as well (undoubtedly a giant in illustrated anatomy but not an illustrator himself), as will Leonardo da Vinci and, sometimes, Max Brödel—arguably the most influential medical illustrator of modern times and the founder of the first graduate school of medical illustration in North America. Needless to say, that doesn't start to cover the rich history of medical illustration, or the omnipresence of illustrations in medical practice, education, the pharmaceutical and surgical technology industries, the medicolegal field, social media, scientific research, and so many other disciplines today.

Medical illustrators can be forgiven a sense of frustration for being so underappreciated. But what makes them really mad is when someone invariably refers to a medical illustration in a slide presentation as a "cartoon." That implies a simplistic divertissement to lighten up an otherwise drab text slide. *Au contraire*—a good illustration doesn't just complement an explanation, it replaces it; clearer than any text

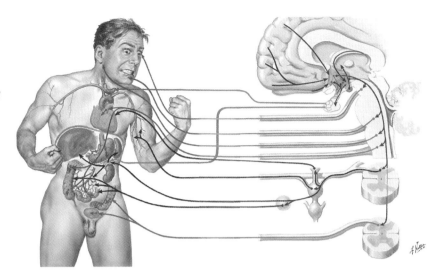

could be, it draws viewers in and helps them understand a difficult concept, a complex anatomic relationship, or an intricate operation.

A Little History

Most humans are visual beings, and many of us like to draw. But medical illustrators are really good at it. And while they tend to have a scientific background, or at least an affinity for the sciences, their genealogy is an artistic one first. A very select few have been great artists *and* great scientists, and one of the greatest was Leonardo da Vinci. Half a century before Vesalius, he had performed countless dissections and sketched his findings in his many notebooks. Da Vinci's drawings of a human fetus in utero, the musculoskeletal anatomy of the trunk, the heart of an ox are all iconic images that are familiar to most of us. Of course, few individuals have had the talent and scientific curiosity of da Vinci. Thus, anatomists, physicians, surgeons, and other scientists since the dawn of modern medicine needed to seek the collaboration of talented artists. This association has endured throughout the centuries, thanks to a combination of shared and complementary qualities.

As medical knowledge grew, illustrators were there to document. The first age of discovery in medicine was the unraveling of human anatomy. Andreas Vesalius, in 1543, published his seminal work, *De Humani Corporis Fabrica* (Of the fabric of the human body), in which he described in detail the skeletal, muscular, and visceral anatomy of a human (Fig. 2).[1] Of course, his work is mostly remembered for its gor-

MedSpeak Illuminated

VIGESIMASECVNDA QVINTI LIBRI FIGVRA·

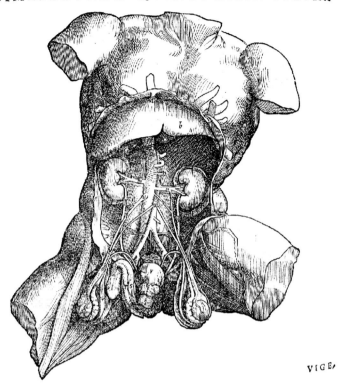

VIGE/

Fig. 2: Andreas Vesalius, *De Humani Corporis Fabrica* (Of the fabric of the human body), 1543, p. 372.

geously accurate illustrations, and his work is so well known because of the invention, exactly a century earlier, of the printing press. In an era when physiology was in its infancy and medical treatments were often painful, sometimes barbaric, and always unscientific, anatomy was the leading medical discipline. Vesalius, Gabriele Fallopio, Govert Bidloo, Xavier Bichat, and William and John Hunter—bridging more than two centuries—all advanced the field of anatomy, and all associated themselves with artists to illustrate their findings.

When, a century after Vesalius, William Harvey described the principles of blood circulation, he used illustrations to explain his findings. And just as the age of anatomic discovery had been documented by artists, the age of physiology required illustrators to disseminate this new medical knowledge. Today, medical illustrators still assist scientists in explaining micro- (rather than macro-) anatomy, down to the cellular, the subcellular, and the molecular. But the last great change in the role of medical illustrators came at the end of the nineteenth century. The discovery of aseptic techniques and anesthesia paved the way for modern surgery. Where medical illustrators had been indispensable in documenting the dissection of the human body, surgeons now sought artists to illustrate their operations. The history of medical illustration in Europe and North America is intimately associated with the rise of visceral, gynecological, and neurosurgery, and the necessity to explain increasingly complex procedures to colleagues and students.

The twentieth century saw an explosion in medical and surgical therapies, ever more complex procedures and interventions fueled by rapidly gained medical knowledge, and all this had to be documented. While we still admire the classic anatomic plates from Vesalius's masterpiece or those of Henry Vandyke Carter in *Gray's Anatomy*, medical illustration today is more readily associated with surgical atlases and scientific articles on innovative interventions.[2]

This is obviously an oversimplification: medical illustration is a subgenre of scientific illustration or, in today's parlance, scientific visualization or SciViz. This very broad field includes any form of graphic representation of biomedical concepts, including microscopic anatomy, molecular structures, biochemical pathways, physiology, and pathophysiology. It also touches on graphic design, page layout, and the best way to give a slide presentation. Scientific visualization itself is no longer limited to two-dimensional illustration. It includes three- and four-dimensional representations, from 3-D printing and physical modeling to time-lapse animations, and from simulation labs to graphic representation of "big data." Any attempt at covering the essence of a topic as rich as scientific illustration is bound to be incomplete. Choices have to be made, and crucial areas will likely be touched upon only superficially or omitted altogether. Rather than going for completeness, what follows is one person's view on the field of medical illustration from the subjective vantage point of clinical surgery and surgical education.

What Is So Special about Medical Illustration?

The ideal attributes of medical illustrators are very similar to those of the best doctors: astute observers, skilled at their craft, and excellent communicators. It is evident that an illustrator must be good at sketching, drawing, and painting, just as a doctor must have a good fund of medical knowledge, and a surgeon must possess fine operating skills. But *great* doctors, like *great* visual artists, are aware of their environment, observe details that others may not pick up on, and see things objectively and without preconceived ideas. Being attuned to

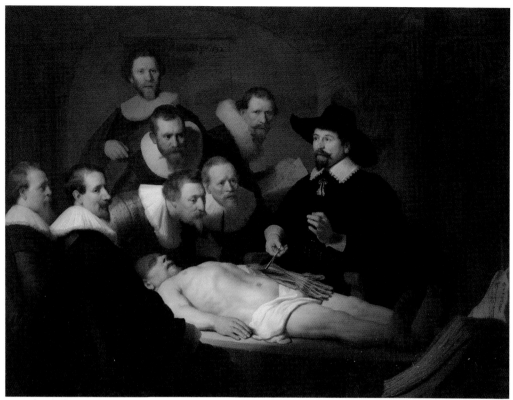

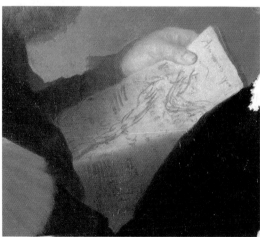

Fig. 3: Rembrandt van Rijn, *De Anatomische Les van Dr. Nicolaes Tulp* (The anatomy lesson of Dr. Nicolaes Tulp), 1632. *Left:* Close-up showing the sheet of paper held by the character to the left of Dr. Tulp. The annotated sketches of the muscles of an extended and a flexed arm are prime examples of the didactic use of medical illustration.

their environment includes an understanding of their audience and the ability to relay information effectively in a comprehensible and accessible way. Throughout history, artists have represented contemporary life, customs, fashions, and the human condition, with its flaws and diseases. Even before artists became medical illustrators, they were interested in anatomy and medicine. Rembrandt van Rijn's *Anatomy Lesson of Dr. Nicolaes Tulp* (Fig. 3) is a prime example of this fascination but hardly the only one. At its base, it is an official group portrait of the famous anatomist and his team, in the same vein as Rembrandt's *The Night Watch,* which immortalized Capt. Frans Banninck Cocq and his company. But the anatomy lesson is much more than a portrait, at least to many of us. It is one of the most famous representations in art of a strictly medical scene. With his right hand, Dr. Tulp is pinching the flexor digitorum muscles of the subject's exposed forearm. With his left hand, he demonstrates the effect of tensing these muscles by flexing his own fingers.

The painting also brings together art, education, and medical illustration. The individual who hangs over the cadaver's head is the only one looking at Dr. Tulp's demonstration of the forearm muscles and tendons—in fact, he seems to stare at the cadaver's hand, anticipating flexion of the fingers; most of the others gaze at a point beyond the dissected arm—a large book in the lower right corner of the painting that some believe to be Vesalius's *De Humani Corporis Fabrica* (although we discern only printed text, they would have stared at one of the beautifully detailed woodcut prints of the atlas).[3] The character immediately to the left of Dr. Tulp holds a sheet of paper with annotated drawings of the muscles of a flexed arm and an extended one: he is using sketches to better understand anatomic relationships, a perfect example of the practical role of medical illustration.

Nicolaes Tulp held the post of praelector in anatomy for the Guild of Surgeons in Amsterdam and later became mayor of the city. In his role at the Guild, he was succeeded by Dr. Jan Deijman, whose anatomy lesson was also immortalized by Rembrandt (see Fig. 97 in chapter 3). One of Tulp's mentees, Frederik Ruysch, is the subject of two anatomic group paintings, one of which may be the first depiction in art of a newborn baby with umbilical cord and placenta still attached—all in vivid colors and remarkably accurate details (Fig. 4). Ruysch's contributions to medical knowledge include the demonstration of the lymphatic system and treatises on teratology.[4] One of his daughters, Rachel Ruysch, was a gifted artist—like her grandfather—and became a celebrated still-life painter.[5] Rachel and Frederik collaborated on dioramas and other projects,[6] but there is no evidence that she illustrated her father's scientific experiments or anatomic dissections. (Her work is now featured alongside *The Night Watch* and Vermeer's *Het Melkmeisje* (The milkmaid) (Fig. 158) in the Rijksmuseum's Eregalerij (Gallery of honor), the first time in the museum's two hundred–year history that a female artist's work is showcased there.[7])

Frederik Ruysch and his artist daughter may have never worked together on medical treatises, but other artists and scientists did.

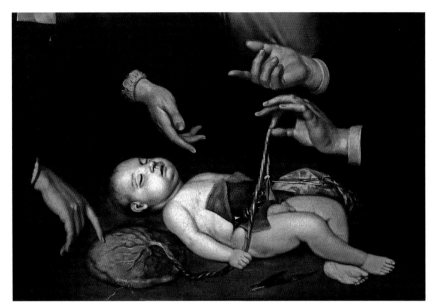

Fig. 4: Jan van Neck, *Anatomische Les van Dr. Frederik Ruysch* (The anatomy lesson of Dr. Frederik Ruysch), circa 1683 (detail).

When renowned anatomist Govert Bidloo needed illustrations for his anatomical atlas, he turned to one of the most notable painters of his day, Gerard de Lairesse, himself a student of Rembrandt's, although he claimed many other influences from Italy and France as well. A century earlier, Vesalius had requested the help of at least one of Titian's disciples, Jan Steven Van Calcar. The sixteenth and seventeenth centuries were marked by anatomic discoveries, and many of the scientists who published their work found similar fruitful associations with artists. This partnership persisted through the age of surgical discovery, and led to the creation of a new field, with its rules, standards, and even its schools—the first of which would become the Department of Art as Applied to Medicine at Johns Hopkins University School of Medicine.[8]

Why Not Photographs?

Before Gutenberg, dissemination of knowledge was limited to direct transmission from teacher to pupil, and any written documents (and images) were painstakingly reproduced by hand, one manuscript at the time. After the invention of the printing press, large-scale production of manuscripts and books became possible, including the reproduction of woodcuts, copper engravings, and lithographs—the only ways to reproduce images for five centuries. Then came photography, an even more faithful reproduction of reality. Of course, early photography was black-and-white and grainy, required long exposure times, and did not rise to the quality and detail of master illustrators. That would certainly explain why, for most of the twentieth century, pen-and-ink or color drawings and paintings remained the most effective and accurate way to document anatomic findings, surgical procedures, medical treatments, and advances in medical research. The quality of photography and videography today, and the ability to digitally optimize these images, should have well surpassed the best artists' work, if all that was required was a faithful reproduction of reality. But medical illustration is something else.

To replace a thousand words, an image must convey the same information in a clear and unequivocal way, which sometimes means deviating from the cold reality. Any concept or idea carries with it an intrinsic, extrinsic, and germane cognitive load. The intrinsic cognitive load is the inherent complexity of a problem. Some ideas are simple to grasp, but most concepts that are worth explaining in detail are not. Whether it is a never-before-done operation that has a high degree of difficulty or risk, or a complicated signaling pathway, there is little we can do to change the idea itself. However, we can streamline the presentation of the concept by focusing on the germane cognitive load—that which *has* to be shown—as it is essential to the entire message; and by eliminating (or minimizing) the extrinsic cognitive load: the extraneous, the superfluous, the details that only distract from the main idea without adding value.[9]

An intraoperative photograph of a cholecystectomy (removal of the gallbladder), for example, may demonstrate all the details of the operative field—the liver, the gallbladder, the adjacent intestines and

Fig. 5: An idealized, lifelike illustration of the abdominal cavity shows organs in their normal relationships but contains too much unnecessary information if the goal is to illustrate the specific details of a surgical procedure.

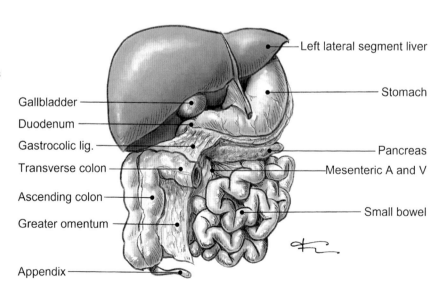

Left lateral segment liver

Stomach

Gallbladder

Duodenum

Gastrocolic lig.

Transverse colon

Ascending colon

Greater omentum

Appendix

Pancreas

Mesenteric A and V

Small bowel

MedSpeak Illuminated

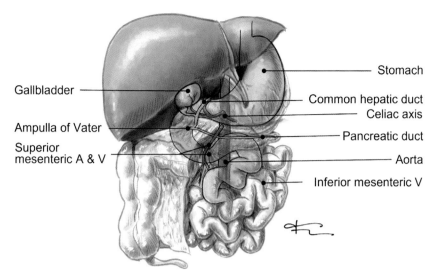

Gallbladder

Ampulla of Vater

Superior
mesenteric A & V

Stomach

Common hepatic duct

Celiac axis

Pancreatic duct

Aorta

Inferior mesenteric V

Fig. 6: Annotations, cutaways (such as the transverse colon to show the small intestine underneath it), and transparency (the aorta and its branches, for example) can add useful details to a medical illustration in ways a photograph alone may not.

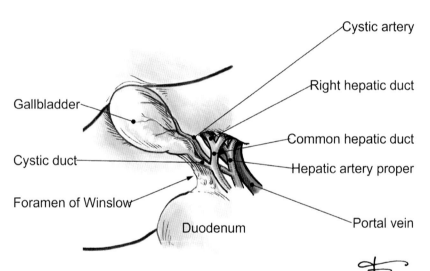

Gallbladder

Cystic duct

Foramen of Winslow

Duodenum

Cystic artery

Right hepatic duct

Common hepatic duct

Hepatic artery proper

Portal vein

Fig. 7: Judicious choice of the viewing angle and omission of extraneous information help the viewer focus on the germane aspects of the gallbladder and biliary anatomy if the goal is to explain the critical aspects of a cholecystectomy.

stomach, the overlying omentum, but it may also show adhesions be-tween the wall of the gallbladder (which may obscure the cystic duct), or any small hematoma caused by bruising with an instrument—de-tails that add clutter and reduce the clarity of the didactic image. An illustration of the abdominal cavity can eliminate the idiosyncrasies and imperfections of the real world, showing a more idealized version of nature (Fig. 5). It can also be annotated, cut away some organs to show others, or demonstrate structures by transparency in ways a photograph alone cannot (Fig. 6). But a truly instructional illustration minimizes structures that are less important in context and draws the eye of the viewer to the task at hand (such as *What are the anatomic* landmarks necessary to safely perform a cholecystectomy?): the cystic duct, the cystic artery, and the common bile duct (Fig. 7). The liver, which takes up a large portion of the abdominal cavity and obstructs the critical portions of the porta hepatis (the area with the ducts and arteries), can be merely hinted at with a few lines to help orient the viewer and situate the action.

Furthermore, the illustrator may find that, in order to show *all* the critical steps of the operation, it may be better to alter the angle of view to expose more of the critical anatomic landmarks. They may also choose to show multiple steps of the operation in the same image, as long as the viewer understands that these are successive rather than simultaneous steps. The artist can show what will be done, what is being done, and what has been done in a single image. The illustrator can add arrows to indicate motion of a structure or an instrument, symbols (like a dotted line and a stylized pair of scissors to indicate where a structure must be divided) (Fig. 8). All these elements constitute a medical illustration, which conveys much more information than even the best of photographs—and often than a full video.[10]

Clearly, medical illustration is as much about communication as it is about reflecting reality. Learning the skills required to become a good medical illustrator is all about observing, analyzing, and communicating. Coincidentally, these are attributes that characterize a good physician too. Paying attention to detail, analyzing the information, and distilling the important points without adding unnecessary detail while considering all the data—all these are critical for doctors as well.[11] As doctors, and certainly as academic physicians, we must also have the skills to convey that information in the clearest possible way—whether to explain to a patient or family, or to teach students and residents.[12] Thus, physicians should not only appreciate medical illustrations (and illustrators) for what they are. They should learn the illustrators' techniques to become better communicators themselves.

Medical Illustration Today

Medical illustration, far from becoming an obsolete discipline with the introduction of photography and videography, has continued

Fig. 8: To optimize its didactic value, a medical illustration can combine anatomic details with classic symbols, like arrows and scissors, and other annotations. Here, a severe stricture of the ureter, as it enters the bladder, caused proximal dilation. The surgeon transected the abnormal ureter just above the narrowing (scissors and dotted line) and swung its proximal end to the contralateral ureter (arrow), where it was anastomosed in an end-to-side fashion.

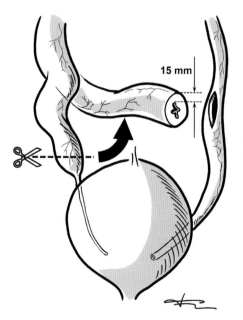

15 mm

to flourish. Technical advances in centuries past were primarily centered around image reproduction: the invention of the printing press first made wide distribution possible, but woodcuts were limited in their versatility and nuance. Copper engravings allowed the use of gray tones (grisaille), and lithography, centuries later, opened the door to color reproduction. Today, digital technology offers limitless possibilities to the artist as well as the publisher: computer-assisted design (CAD) and affordable graphic programs allow the enlightened amateur to produce professional-looking illustrations, and the professional to create masterworks in a fraction of the time it would have taken in the analog world—if they could have been created at all. In addition to the didactic value of scientific illustration, the field has gone in at least three new directions that reflect our times. The first is exemplified by the origins of Frank Netter's artistic career. He was approached by the pharmaceutical company CIBA (now a subsidiary of Novartis) to create a full-color anatomic illustration of the heart to be used for an advertisement for the drug digitalis. Its success was such that CIBA commissioned additional plates, and that project eventually led to his eight-volume opus, the *CIBA Collection of Medical Illustrations*. Advertisement has relied on medical illustrations ever since, enticing physicians to prescribe a company's products using glossy pamphlets with full-color images. These print ads gradually made way for television commercials, adding 3-D and animation to the armamentarium of medical illustrators. Advertising is a reality of modern American society; lawsuits are another. A growing branch of medical illustration is now devoted to legal work in civil court, often for the plaintiff. A well-crafted, vividly realistic illustration of someone's injuries or painful, serial operations is much more evocative than a dry recitation of medical records. While the goal is to shock, or at least to move, the principles of a good court illustration are no different than those of classic medical illustration: to convey a message as clearly as possible, emphasizing the important factors while minimizing extraneous or distracting details.

The most recent trend in medical illustration is its adaptation to social media. Increasingly, medical breakthroughs or incremental research discoveries are announced by scientific journals or societies with short posts and simple, flashy graphics that catch the reader's attention. Many have deplored society's trend toward "dumbing down" and decreasing attention span—and on the surface, it would appear that the best way to get clicks on Twitter, for example, is to post a picture (see also TL; DR; the tongue-in-cheek acronym to indicate loss of interest—"Too Long; Didn't Read"). In reality, these "infographics" may play a more fundamentally helpful role. In an era when more and more information is available and it is impossible to read everything in one's field, these catchy images serve as a quick and efficient shorthand to help us decide whether an article is relevant or interesting. The habit of scanning a scientific article for relevance has always existed: traditionally, that was the role of the abstract. Every scientific paper opens with a short summary of the work, from a short introduction or background, through methods and results, to a brief conclusion. The clinician, scholar, or scientist knows enough about the topic to decide from the abstract if the paper itself is worth reading in detail. Today, the abstract has been replaced by a tweet and, more recently, by a new form of communication: the visual abstract. These are typically three frames containing graphic elements and icons, minimal text, the title of the paper and some form of branding (color scheme, font, logo) that rapidly identifies the journal or society that advertises the study. This is medical illustration at its most basic: the combination of graphic arts and text to convey a clear message, understandable by all.

New Competition: Diagnostic Imaging

Medical illustration survived the photographic age because it was better able to cut to the chase, to weed out the excess information offered by a truthful rendition of the visible world. In the last century, a new form of medical visualization has emerged: the visual rendition of the invisible world. When Wilhelm Roentgen produced a radiograph of his wife's hand, complete with radio-opaque wedding band, it was the first time that people could see inside the body. There was the prospect of understanding the inner anatomy and inner human workings without the need to dissect or operate. But just like early photography, early X-ray images were grainy, crude, and often difficult to interpret. The principle of early radiography is similar to that of early photography: activation of silver particles by light or X-rays, turning them black by developing the plate. Radiographs are therefore black and white and do not reflect the natural colors of tissues. Similarly, when ultrasonography became widespread in medicine, in the 1970s, they were gray-scale images as the reflected sound waves emitted by the probe captured the differences in tissue density. For the initiated, these austere pictures were very clear and immensely helpful. For everyone else, they were often undecipherable and rarely inspiring. Medical illustrations, however, could be vivid, colorful, exciting—and definitely more accessible to students and the lay public.

In recent decades, spectacular advances in diagnostic imaging technology have allowed us to move from two-dimensional radiographs to three-dimensional images (computerized axial tomography, or CT scan, magnetic resonance imaging (MRI) and 3-D ultrasound). Digital capture of cross-sectional body slices can now be reconstructed to look like veritable three-dimensional objects that can even be colorized, rivaling the most intricate illustrations. Moreover, postproduction manipulation of the images can achieve what medical illustration can but photography can't: eliminate extraneous information by cutting out layers or less relevant organs to make the image more didactic.[13] In some cases, it is almost impossible to tell the difference between an artist's rendition of internal organs and a computer-generated volume rendering of a CT scan of the same subject.[14] No matter how sophisticated, however, the radiograph reflects the subject faithfully: any distracting imperfections, motion artifacts, or technical glitches will show up as well (Fig. 9), whereas the medical illustrator can idealize the image to fit the need (Fig. 10). These two disciplines also have different (if sometimes overlapping) purposes: diagnostic imaging serves to establish a diagnosis in a particular patient, while medical illustration often explains in more general terms. This doesn't mean that they can't collaborate, and modern illustrators gladly use photographs *and* diagnostic imaging to enhance their own work.[15]

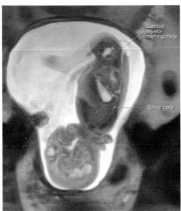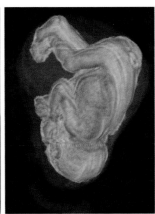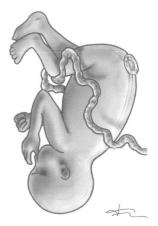

Left and center: Fig. 9: Modern diagnostic imaging, such as MRI, can offer exquisite details of even the smallest structures, such as a fetus with a spinal cord defect (*left*). However, even the best postacquisition manipulation of the image is flawed because of technical limitations, motion artifacts, and other imperfections (volume rendering of the same image, *center*).

Right: Fig. 10: Artist's interpretation of the MRI image in Fig. 9, maintaining anatomic accuracy while eliminating extraneous or distracting details.

A Beautiful Friendship

Visual artists may care about the esthetic of their work or the faithful reproduction of nature. Medical illustration, while drawing from art, is much more than a pretty picture or a verisimilar one. Medical illustrators aspire to observe, analyze, and explain in the clearest way possible.[16] The perfect illustration, then, provides an esthetically pleasing end result of a carefully planned explanation, and is best achieved when doctor and artist collaborate closely.[17] This is also why physicians can become better doctors by learning about medical illustration.

We are visual beings, and to borrow from *New Yorker* illustrator Christoph Niemann, we all understand a common language without ever having learned it, without even knowing it: the visual language.[18] This is why all doctors draw. We may not all be Frank Netters, but we have all, at some point in our practice, drawn out what we were trying to explain to a patient or a family, to a medical student or a resident, or to colleagues. Some doctors are true artists and gifted illustrators (Frank Netter was a physician; Dr. Jean-Martin Charcot drew caricatures; and Harvey Cushing, founder of modern neurosurgery, was an artist in his own right); others are less adept, but wouldn't mind getting better.[19] Simple principles of light, shadows, perspective, and composition can dramatically enhance a drawing and make it easier to understand. Moreover, spending the necessary time to consider how to illustrate an operation, a treatment, or a pathway, deciding on which steps of an operation to show or which details of a cellular cascade to focus on, forces us to think about the procedure or the reaction itself. It forces us to formulate an idea, and it may help us understand it better.[20] As the saying goes, "If you can't explain it simply, you don't understand it well enough." This applies to the creation of the perfect medical illustration too. And it is relevant for both the physician and the medical illustrator: understanding the subject and knowing what has to be emphasized and what can be omitted are important to both.

There is a recent trend in medical education to take students to museums of fine art, and have them observe and describe paintings, the better to hone their observational, diagnostic, and even empathic skills.[21] This, in turn, makes them more caring providers: it teaches them to focus on small but potentially meaningful details; to read body language and facial expressions; and to see what is there rather than to assume. Amy Herman, founder of The Art of Perception, Inc. and author of *Visual Intelligence: Sharpen Your Perception, Change Your Life* uses these techniques to teach law enforcement officers, physicians, and many other professionals to do just that, whether to make our airports safer or become better team leaders. In her book and seminars, she focuses on observation of art and life.[22] As physicians, we can go one step further: we can learn to observe, analyze, and explain by learning to draw (better). Rather than describing a situation, a syndrome, or a finding, we can visualize it. We can learn from our colleagues in medical illustration, not to replace them (we still need them to create polished and professional illustrations), but to become better observers and communicators as we explain medical situations to patients, families, students, and colleagues. And most professional medical illustrators will say that their work can be greatly facilitated if the doctors who request their services are themselves better visual communicators. This book is not an instructional manual on drawing and illustration. It does, however, show the tight relationship between visual arts, medicine, and communication—just like Rick Blaine and Captain Renaud in *Casablanca,* doctors and medical illustrators throughout history have enjoyed "a beautiful friendship."

Chapter 1

History of Medical Illustration

Artists have, for centuries, been witness to society's changes, including the changes in medical knowledge and practice. Keen observers, they have accurately depicted health and disease in manners both obvious and hidden. That does not automatically make them medical illustrators, however. What differentiates art in medicine from medical illustration is a sense of purpose: the ultimate goal of a scientific illustrator is to teach, to explain, to communicate. No matter how beautiful an illustration may be—and many are true works of art—its didactic value is what matters most. Skilled scientific illustrators know what needs to be explained, and build from there, often in collaboration with the physician or scientist whose work is being highlighted. The final illustration impresses not only for its artistic value but for the clarity of its message.

Seeing Is Believing

What follows here is not an exhaustive catalog of medical illustration through the ages. Rather, it is an attempt to situate it within the broader field of medicine; to show its role as witness of the advances in anatomic knowledge, medical discovery, and surgical innovation in the last six centuries; and to describe how it became a bona fide profession that is now more relevant than ever. Humans are visual beings. Vision is the most important of our senses. We can fool our other senses by altering images: the McGurk effect describes how the perception of the spoken word can be changed if the person who is speaking seems to mouth different consonants.[1] Food can taste differently, depending on its color (a steak colored with green dye will taste bitter) or the color of the plate it is served on. In medicine, as in many other disciplines, visual examination is paramount, from visual inspection during a physical exam to graphic representation of a physiologic concept, a pharmacological reaction, or a surgical procedure. We certainly use our other senses as well, or at least we used to when diagnostic modalities were more limited. Before chemical analysis of urine and blood were possible, skilled physicians could glean a lot from examining not only the color and turbidity of urine but the smell and even the taste of it (sweet-tasting urine was a sign that the patient was spilling sugar, indicating diabetes). Sounds are important in medicine, too—auscultation of the lungs or the heart, detection of bowel sounds, or percussion of a hollow or fluid-filled body cavity. These are more difficult skills to acquire and much harder to teach than visual skills, however, and they have become less essential for the clinician thanks to the development of sophisticated diagnostic tools, including diagnostic imaging.

Images are often more helpful than words (as the adage says, "Show, don't tell"). Lengthy descriptions of a process, an operation, or an anatomic relationship are much harder to grasp than an illustration of the same.[2] Furthermore, images transcend languages and literacy. This was true centuries ago, when illiteracy was more prevalent, and still is true today, not in the least because our specialized jargon, or "Med-Speak," has become more inscrutable to the uninitiated. In medicine and other life sciences, images have always played an important role in the dissemination of knowledge. Their role has changed through history and has paralleled medical and scientific knowledge.

The Prehistory of Medical Illustration

Prehistoric imagery is rare, but cave paintings have been preserved or discovered, such as those in Lascaux in the Dordogne (France), and Altamira and El Pindal (northern Spain). In the Pindal cave, a peculiar outline of a mammoth was found with the imprint of a heart in the animal's chest. According to some experts, it was an early how-to instruction drawing on the most effective way to kill a mammoth (Fig. 11).[3] Dating back approximately fifteen thousand years ago, it is arguably one of the oldest examples of scientific illustration in the

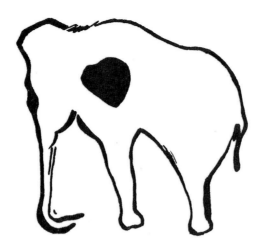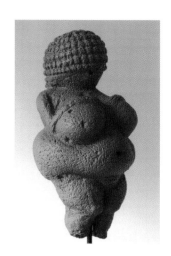

Fig. 11: Henri (Abbé) Breuil (1877–1961), Magdalenian representation of a mammoth, Upper Paleolithic. Reproduction of a cave painting in El Pindal, Spain. Depiction of the heart inside a mammoth may have been an instruction on where to strike most effectively—a prehistoric form of medical illustration? (Wellcome Images, licensed under CC BY 4.0.)

Fig. 12: Venus of Willendorf (Austria, 23,000 years BC), likely meant as a fertility amulet. (Photograph by Bjørn Christian Tørrissen, licensed under CC BY-SA 4.0.)

world. Of course, we do not know the exact meaning or purpose of these cave paintings, and it is difficult to consider any of these images as "medical" in the modern sense of the word. (An equally plausible explanation is that the heart-shaped spot on the pachyderm's thorax is a bloodied hunting wound.)

We have been aware of our health and anatomy throughout history, and have entertained explanations for many disease manifestations, their origins, and their possible cures. Before the age of discovery, superstitions and the supernatural were significant driving forces behind life's mysteries. Even older than the cave paintings of mammoth hearts are the so-called Venus figurines, the most famous of which is the Venus, or Woman, of Willendorf (Fig. 12), dating back to 23,000 BC. These female statuettes exhibit exaggerated breasts and hips and protuberant bellies, suggesting that they may have been used as fertility amulets.[4] These, too, could be considered prehistoric forms of medical illustration depicting pregnancy. Many ancient civilizations were known to possess some degree of medical and surgical knowledge. The funerary stele of Pharaonic priest Ruma (thirteenth-century BC) shows him with a thin, shortened leg and deformed foot, believed to depict the ravages of poliomyelitis.[5] Egyptian hieroglyphs have been found that describe circumcision (Fig. 13), lancing of abscesses, skull trepanation, and drainage of hematomas. Trepanation, in particular, is a remarkably consistent practice throughout history and across many civilizations (Fig. 14).[6] Trephines, or trepans, are devices used to burr a hole through the scalp and the skull in order to relieve a patient of symptoms and diseases. The exact nature of the conditions that were treated in such manner is of course unclear, but ancient civilizations would have known that head injuries, whether iatrogenic or accidental, were often lethal.

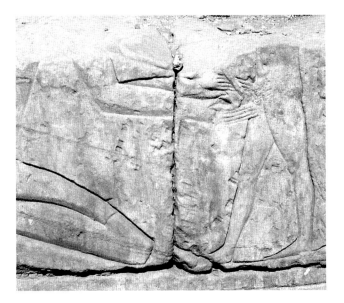

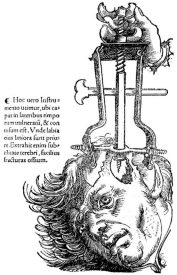

❡ Hoc uero Inſtru⸗
mento utimur, ubi ca⸗
put in lateribus tempo
rum uulneratū, & con
tuſum eſt. Vnde labia
eius latiora ſunt prio⸗
re. Extrahit enim ſub⸗
tilitate terebri, facilius
fracturas oſſium.

There is ample evidence that these trepanations were often deliberate, and that patients would have survived the insult (witnessed by evidence of bone healing around the trepanation wound, suggesting survival for years or even decades). One can imagine that the simple drainage of a subdural hematoma would have been life-saving in the right hands.[7] Without treatment, these blunt injuries lead to compression of the brain, seizures, coma, and death. The occasional successes with the surgical cure of traumatic seizures may have emboldened some to offer craniotomy for less clear indications, such as epilepsy and madness, sometimes referred to as "removing the stone of folly" (Fig. 15).[8]

It may seem strange that of all the possible surgical interventions our ancestors would have mastered, skull trepanation is one of the most ubiquitous. In the absence of sterile conditions, sophisticated instruments, knowledge of pathology and physiology, and any meaningful medication (never mind the lack of anesthesia), attempting brain surgery would have been a daunting concept. Of course, most traces of any surgical interventions on soft organs and body parts would have been erased with the decay of tissues. The only structures that have been preserved are bones, with their wounds and, in some cases, their healing scars. It could suggest that ancient civilizations were more adept at other interventions as well, but these have not left any traces. The finding of healing burr holes in ancient skulls is corroborated by countless illustrations (engravings, paintings, and sculptures): while most of these images are merely documenting daily life, at least some of them, like the woodcut in (Fig. 14), can be regarded as medical illustrations in the true sense of a didactic, how-to manual.

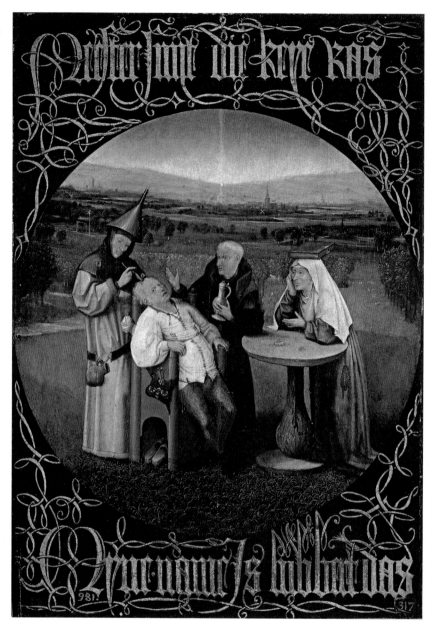

Medical illustration is a relatively young profession, but so is modern medicine as its practice was truly formalized only a few centuries ago. Healing arts in ancient civilizations was closely intertwined with religion, myth, and superstition, as humans tried to rationalize what could not yet be explained. The gods were invoked to produce a good harvest, guarantee fertility, or ward off death and disease. People would put their faith in priests for all spiritual and physical problems. The profession of medicine developed much later. Until the Renaissance, the field of the healing arts was shared by doctors, barber-surgeons, nurses, and midwives, each with their well-defined realm.[9]

Barber-Surgeons

Long before scientific discovery paved the way for the experimental basis of surgery, anesthesia, and asepsis, surgery was a purely skill-based occupation. One did not need to know much to be a good surgeon—one needed to be fast and accurate, and good with sharp objects. Naturally, someone who could offer a close shave without nicking the customer could use his knife skills for other purposes as well, such as lancing a boil or cauterizing a wound. They could swiftly pull a rotten tooth, providing immediate relief. Speed and showmanship were important attributes, and a good surgeon was also an entertaining one, playing to the masses during carnivals and fairs. David Teniers, Frans Hals, and other seventeenth-century painters have famously captured these scenes, where dentists offer their services to the people, amid "low-brow" entertainment, too much food, and too much wine (Fig. 16). Barber-surgeons practiced their skills—draining a hydrocele, lancing a wound (Fig. 17), or scraping a hemorrhoid—procedures that required little knowledge but a steady hand. If the treatment was bloody, or foul-smelling pus gushed from the boil, so much the better: at a time

Fig. 16: Jan Steen, *De Tandentrekker* (The tooth-puller), 1651.

Fig. 17: David Teniers the Younger, *A Surgeon Lancing a Grimacing Man's Shoulder,* 1678. Engraving by Jacob Coelemans, 1703. (Wellcome Images, licensed under CC BY 4.0.)

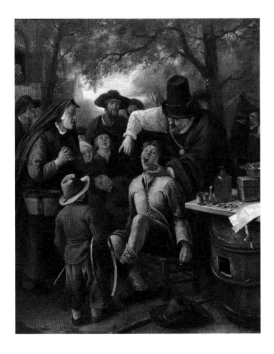

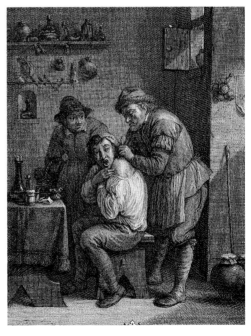

when few diseases were understood, let alone curable, only barber-surgeons and dentists could offer instant and spectacular relief, and they reveled in the sheer brutality of it. Gore was a source of pride for barber-surgeons, and bloody bandages became their signature. Thus, the red-and-white spiral barber's pole was born, or so goes one of the theories behind its origin.

Surgeons honed their skills in peace time, but their true moment to shine was on the battlefield. Following a military tradition that continues until today (surgical advances have been made after every modern war, from the treatment of shock and gunshot wounds in the Vietnam War to the management of blast injuries in the many conflicts in the Middle East and Northern Ireland),[10] combat medicine

Fig. 18: *A Surgeon Treating a Thigh Wound.* Detail from a fresco found at Pompeii, submerged AD 79. (Wellcome Images, licensed under CC BY 4.0.)

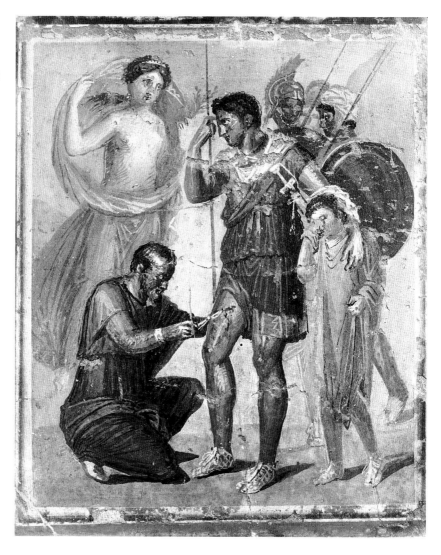

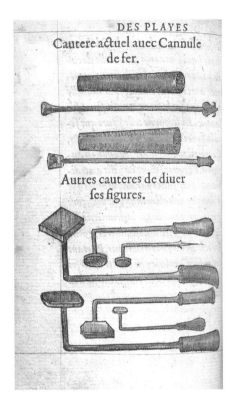

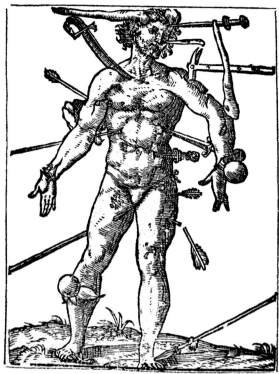

has been well documented through the ages. Whether early images of war injuries were meant to be educational rather than simply figurative is, of course, speculation. It is striking, however, that many of the minor surgical procedures depicted in Greek, Roman, and Egyptian art relate to combat trauma (Fig. 18). Eventually, documenting military injuries made way for cataloging them. Ambroise Paré, a pioneer of modern trauma surgery, was a field surgeon.[11] His twenty-six-volume *Oeuvres,* published in 1575, summarizes his experience as "Premier chirurgien du roi" (first surgeon of the king), most of it acquired on the battlefield (Fig. 19).[12]

A particular type of illustration, popular in Europe in the fourteenth through seventeenth centuries, is clearly meant as an instructional manual. It is referred to as "wound man" (Fig. 20), a representation of what appears to be the unluckiest man in the world. In reality, it is a single illustration of every type of penetrating injury one might have encountered on the battlefield. As far as we understand them, they were used by army doctors to treat the wounded.[13] As with the earlier examples of "medical" illustration, many of these were unique specimens, since they often predate the invention of

Fig. 19: Ambroise Paré, Illustration of a common cautery with iron cannula (*top*) and other cauteries of various shapes (*bottom*), in *La Méthode Curatrice des Playes, et Fractures de la Teste Humaine. Avec Pourtraits des Instruments Nécessaires pour la Curation d'Icelles* (The treatment method of wounds and fractures of the human head. With illustrations of the instruments required for their treatment), 1561. (Wellcome Images, licensed under CC BY 4.0.)

Fig. 20: William Clowes, Wound-man illustration, woodcut, sixteenth century. This seemingly unlucky subject demonstrates all the possible wounds and weapons one may encounter on the battlefield. (Hi-Story / Alamy Stock Photo.)

the printing press. They would have been copied by hand, and some may be found as part of the illuminations of medieval manuscripts.

Serious Doctors

Barber-surgeons and battlefield medics were sought after for their technical skills. "Serious" doctors, however, did not deign to deal directly with blood and pus, or get their hands otherwise dirty. Theirs was a profession that grew out of observation and reasoning: they sought to understand the human condition and humans' place in the world. They were often philosophers as well, were fluent in Latin and Greek, and had broader interests that included literature, poetry, or astronomy. While religion and superstition gradually made way for a more scientific approach, early physicians lacked the rigorous methods of scientific experimentation and the sophisticated tools to come to a correct diagnosis. Without laboratory tests or radiographs, early physicians had to rely on their clinical acumen and observational skills, barely helped by the few diagnostic tools they had—physical examination, and in particular palpation of the pulse and "analysis" of bodily fluids, such as phlegm or urine. The seventeenth-century artists Frans van Mieris, Gerrit Dou, Jan Steen, and others in Holland or England gave us a series of paintings showing the doctor taking a patient's pulse (Fig. 21). The composition of these works of art are all similar—the clear

Fig. 21: Jan Steen, *De Zieke Vrouw* (The sick woman), circa 1665.

Fig. 22: Samuel Van Hoogstraten, *The Bleekzuchtige Dame* The anemic lady), circa 1667.

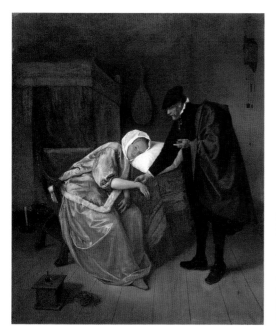

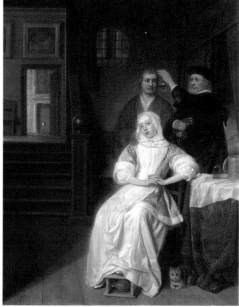

hierarchy, the importance and noble stance of the physician, center stage, surrounded by the patient's family members. Often the patient is a woman, and in at least one painting, she is clearly pale (Fig. 22). Anemia could be due to poor nutrition and low iron concentrations in the blood (so-called ferriprive anemia). It is more common in women than in men, in part because of monthly menstrual blood loss. The condition increases the heart rate as the heart must pump faster to deliver the same amount of hemoglobin-bound oxygen despite a low concentration of red blood cells. Thus, a fast, thready pulse would suggest anemia (and low blood pressure)—an erudite diagnosis, even if its true pathophysiology (or its treatment) eluded the doctor. Examining a patient's urine was another common diagnostic tool—it was easily obtained, and some conditions could be correlated with abnormal findings in the urine: cystitis (bladder infection) would produce pyuria (pus in the urine, rendering it cloudy and foul-smelling); kidney or bladder stones could produce blood in the urine; and fever and sweating, combined with poor hydration and fluid losses from vomiting and diarrhea, would produce dark, concentrated urine in patients who had a viral or bacterial enteritis. So few were the diagnostic options to the seventeenth-century physician that he used all his senses to deduce a diagnosis. He would consider the color of the urine, the smell, and even the taste: sweet urine meant spilled sugar (glucosuria), one of the first signs of diabetes mellitus (literally *flow of honey* in Greek). Urinalysis was an integral part of the limited diagnostic armamentarium of the physician, so much so that St. Cosmas, patron saint of doctors and brother of St. Damian, patron of pharmacists,[14] is often portrayed with a urine flask (Fig. 23). (More on saints' attributes and the relationship with medical illustration later—see chapter 5.)

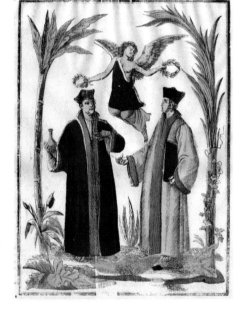

Fig. 23: St. Cosmas and St. Damian, patron saints of physicians and pharmacists. Note the urine flask in St. Cosmas's right hand, symbol of physicians. Image d'Epinal (1796) Color lithograph. (Bibliothèques Médiathèques de Metz, France.)

Because of the contemplative activities of "medical doctors" (as opposed to barber-surgeons, whose trade was much more hands-on and visual), medical instruction relied more on the word than the image. Nevertheless, a few proto-medical illustrations subsist—visual charts to help the bedside physician. To help the physician interpret the examination of a patient's urine, for example, some textbooks offered easy-to-use color charts, complete with all possible hues and degrees of clarity, and their diagnostic equivalent (Fig. 24).

With the creation of the first medical schools in Europe, doctors—who studied anatomy, biology, and philosophy—gradually increased their knowledge of the human body and its functions. Medicinal herbs and plants became available as trade with other parts of the world increased, and pharmacology developed into a growing medical spe-

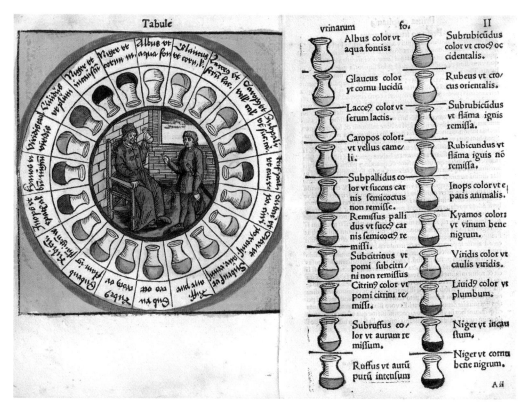

Fig. 24: Ulrich Pinder, Speculum videndi urinas hominum (Visual chart of human urine samples), 1506, in *Epiphanie Medicorum* (Doctors' revelations). The chart describes the color of urine samples as they compare to well-known substances: for example, the top sample in the wheel (*top left on the opposing table*) describes the urine as Albus color ut aqua fontis (white, like fountain water); the one immediately to the right is Subrubicudus color ut crocus occidentalis (reddish yellow, like saffron). (LUNA: Folger Digital Image Collection. Public Domain.)

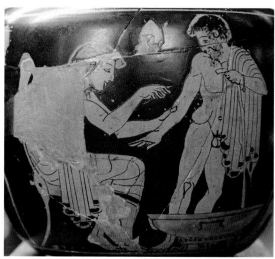

Fig. 25: Clinic Painter, circa 475 BC, Aryballos (oil flask) decorated with a physician treating a patient by bloodletting. (Photograph by Marie-Lan Nguyen, licensed under CC BY 3.0.)

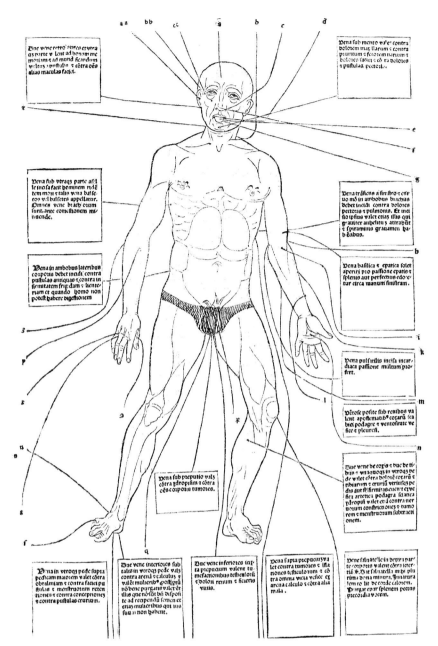

Fig. 26: *Aderlassman* (Bloodletting man), in *Fasciculus Medicinae* (Collection of medical texts) (Germany), 1491. The illustration shows a "bloodletting man" with anatomic descriptions of the best veins to incise, depending on the desired outcome. For example, the vena basilica (basilic vein in the antecubital fossa), also called "hepatic vein" in the illustration, would be accessed to treat "hepatic and splenic passions," a reference to two of the four natural humors, bile and atrabile, whose origins are the liver and the spleen, respectively.

cialty. While doctors could start thinking about treating their patients, they were not ready to get their hands dirty. Few treatments were at their disposal, but even those were usually not delivered by the physicians themselves. Bloodletting and the application of leeches, believed to rid the body of bad humors, had been a practice since antiquity (Fig. 25).[15] The *Aderlassman* (German for *bloodletting man*) in (Fig. 26), a cousin of wound man, shows practitioners where to find the

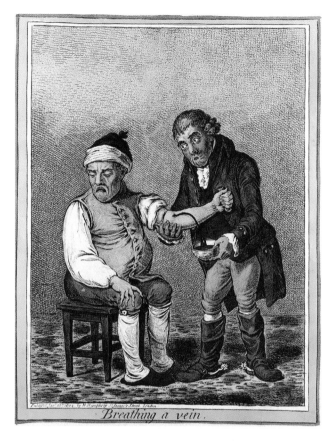

Fig. 27: James Gillray, *Breathing a Vein*, 1804. Note the bloodletting stick in the patient's left hand. The squeeze and a tourniquet made bleeding easier. (Wellcome Images, licensed under CC BY 4.0.)

best spots to draw blood. The illustration also indicates the various benefits of specific bloodletting.[16] Bleeding the basilic vein, in the antecubital fossa, helps to treat "hepatic passion," referring to the liver, where bile (one of the four humors) originates. Too much bile renders the patient "choleric" (from the Greek for *bile, chole* [χολή], which is also the root of cholecystitis—inflammation of the gallbladder and choledochal—of the common bile duct). According to this illustration, bleeding the same vein also treats "splenic passion:" the spleen was allegedly the source of black bile, or "a(n)trabile," better known in its Greek form of *melena chole* (μέλαινα χολή) or melancholy. Humorism (explaining various conditions by an imbalance of the four humors) had been largely disproved by the seventeenth century, but the sanguine (blood), phlegmatic (phlegm), choleric (bile), and melancholic (black bile) temperaments have persisted in our common vocabulary. *Spleen* even made it as a word to describe the generalized melancholy and disillusionment of the early nineteenth century, also referred to as *mal du siècle* (sickness of the century).

Bloodletting was usually performed by incising a forearm vein and letting the blood flow into a cup. Blood flow was enhanced by a tour-

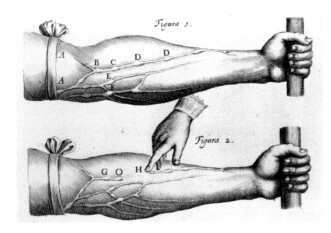

Fig. 28: William Harvey, *Exercitatio Anatomica de Motu Cordis et Sanguinis, in Animalibus* (An anatomical exercise on the motion of the heart and blood in living beings), more commonly called *De motu cordis* (The workings of the heart), 1628: his seminal work, in which he deduces that arterial blood is pumped by the heart, and venous blood returns to the heart to be pumped to the lungs for oxygenation (and not through invisible pores between the left and right ventricles, as Galen had hypothesized). Figure 1 shows engorgement of the forearm veins after a proximal tourniquet has been applied. In Figure 2, the finger of the observer milks the blood toward the subject's wrist (from O to H), and the vein remains empty, suggesting that blood flows unidirectionally from distal to central. Note the tourniquet and bloodletting stick.

niquet and having the patient squeeze a stick (Fig. 27). It is believed that the early symbol for barber-surgeons, and later for barbers, was that stick or pole, topped by a cup or basin (symbolizing the receptacle in which leeches were kept). The corresponding cup at the bottom of the barber's pole represents the basin in which blood was collected. (As mentioned earlier, the red-and-white stripes on the pole might represent bloody bandages, although none of these origin stories are entirely satisfactory.)

That squeezing stick is also pictured in the landmark treatise by William Harvey, *De motu cordis,* in which he first describes the blood circulation—a beautiful early example of simple, effective medical illustration (Fig. 28). More than "pretty pictures," the figures elegantly demonstrate a phenomenon that would otherwise require a very long explanation. This is how Roberto Bolli describes the experiment, carried out on the veiny forearms of muscular farm workers:[17] "[William Harvey] put a tourniquet around the arm and tried to empty the veins with his finger. He noticed that the veins would always fill from the distal to the proximal part of the arm—not vice versa, indicating that blood flows from the hand toward the shoulder. He thus concluded that the blood in the veins always flowed toward the heart."

Instead of a direct incision into the vein, blood could also be teased out by scarification (placing a series of more superficial scratches on the forearm) and vacuum aspiration of blood into previously heated glass cups, a practice that is still used in various places around the world today. Bleeding, cupping, and leech application were the purview of lay practitioners, often women (Fig. 29).

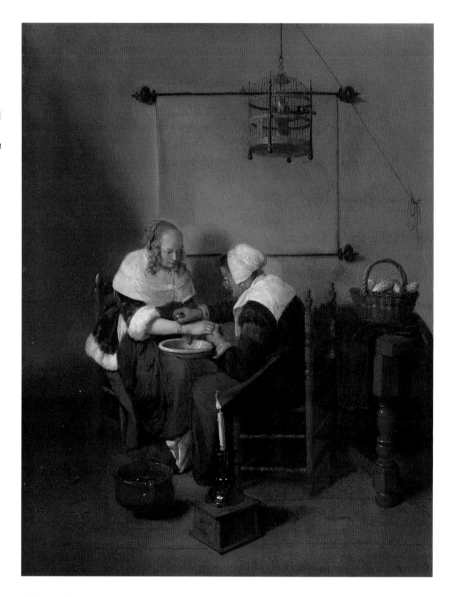

Fig. 29: Quiringh van Brekelenkam, *De Kopster* (The bloodletting), 1660. The skin has been scratched (scarification), and a vacuum cup is applied to draw the blood out.

Obstetrics

Assisting in pregnancy and childbirth was also a woman's job. Midwifery is probably the truly oldest profession, and men did not become involved in obstetrics until the late eighteenth century. Well before medical practices were topics of visual art—indeed, before the invention of the printing press—there were plenty of representations of childbirth, with midwives or doulas in attendance. Similar to wound man and bloodletting man, anatomical figurines of pregnant women with removable internal organs, uterus, and fetus were prevalent in Europe in the Middle Ages, and likely aimed at helping midwives

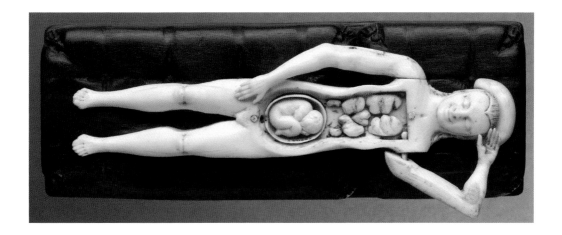

(Fig. 30). Treatises of midwifery are not known before the sixteenth century and would not have been particularly helpful: since childbirth was not the purview of doctors until the eighteenth century, didactic figurines would have been much more effective than written text to illiterate midwives.[18]

Except for puerperal care, the treatment of peripheral wounds, lancing of boils, and pulling of teeth (as well as the occasional skull trepanation), medical practice (and knowledge) in Europe was extremely limited in the first thirteen centuries of the Common Era. The pursuit of medical knowledge was thriving in other parts of the world, however. Large numbers of intricately illustrated manuscripts from Japan and China have survived to this day. These works demonstrate some advanced understanding of anatomy and physiology, knowledge that was inaccessible to Europeans. Western scientists and physicians can be excused for claiming they discovered the principles of respiration, blood flow (William Harvey, 1628), or genetics (Georg Mendel, 1865), unaware that scientists in the East beat them to it by many centuries. The Fertile Crescent, encompassing Asia Minor, the Middle East, and parts of North Africa, was also an intellectually fertile region in the first millennium at a time when scientific curiosity was dormant in the West. Great scholars were physicians, philosophers, mathematicians, biologists, and astronomers. Their writings were not only influential in their time but filled the intellectual void in Europe. The most famous of all was Aelius Galenus, or Galen of Pergamon, who lived in the second century. Pergamon, now Bergama, is in Asia Minor, current-day Turkey—it was part of the Eastern portion of the Roman Empire. Galen is considered the most important physician of his era and one of the most influential scientists of all time. His theories were strengthened by his experimental approach to medicine and anatomy and were the prevailing canon for more than twelve centuries. His teachings in anatomy, in particular, became the established doctrine and were based on meticulous dissections and autopsies.[19] Unfortunately, these were animal dissections (predominantly dogs, pigs, and cattle), which, while generally helpful in understanding mammalian physiology, introduced major flaws in his teachings of human anatomy. No original writings survived, and it is not known whether he ever had his treatises illustrated. He was widely copied, however, and many apocryphal works were written (and later published), perpetuating his teachings. Add to that the rigidity of religious dogma and the intolerance of the church, and Galen's medical theories, right or wrong, remained unchallenged until the middle of the sixteenth century.[20] Anatomic inaccuracies were not the only problems with Galenic medicine. His views on physiology and pathophysiology were heavily influenced by Hippocrates's beliefs in the role of the four humors (blood, phlegm, yellow bile, and black bile), paralleling the four elements (earth, water, wind, and fire).[21] Without the ability to observe internal physiologic processes, much had to be assumed based on observation of an inanimate body. He therefore professed that the venous and arterial circulations were physically separate (one containing bright red blood, the other dark blood). Not believing that much blood could flow through the pulmonary circulation, he believed instead that dark (venous) blood passed from the right side of the heart through invisible pores (the term *microscopic* did not yet exist) in the septum into the left chambers of the heart, where it was mixed with "pneuma" (air) to become bright, arterial blood.[22] It was Ibn al-Nafis, the famous Arabic physician and polymath from Damascus and Egypt, who, in the thirteenth century challenged Galen's theory in his "Commentary on Anatomy in Avicenna's Canon," in which he describes how dark blood flows to the lungs to be exposed to air ("heated"), and returns to the heart as bright red blood.[23] (Avicenna, or Ibn Sina, is considered by many to be the founder of modern medicine; he preceded al-Nafis by some two hundred years.[24] An ardent follower of Galen, Avicenna helped propagate Galen's theories and even embellished them a little. In commenting on Avicenna's canon, al-Nafis was really refuting Galen's beliefs.)

Evidence of Ibn al-Nafis's teaching resurfaced only at the beginning of the twentieth century, rightfully attributing the discovery of the pulmonary circulation to him rather than to the Western scientists who came centuries later[25]—Michael Servetus (in 1553), Realdo Colombo (1559), and, most notably, William Harvey, who with his illustrated *De motu cordis* in 1628 had been widely credited as the "first," possibly demonstrating the power of medical illustration (see Fig. 28).

The power of illustrations is also found in the work of Mansur ibn Muhammad ibn Ilyas, a Persian scholar and physician. His treatise contains the earliest known full-page anatomical illustrations from the Islamic world.[26] (Before that, Galen's anatomical writings were sometimes illustrated with schematic diagrams rather than detailed anatomic images. Whether this was out of deference to aniconism, the prohibition of portraying living beings in Muslim law, is speculative.) *Mansur's Anatomy* consists of six chapters, each illustrated with a full-page anatomic diagram (Fig. 31).

The historic link between detailed anatomic knowledge and human dissections is difficult to establish.[27] Christian and Muslim faiths did not condone autopsies, although Muslim scholars praised the study of anatomy as a way to demonstrate the wisdom of God. Some scholars

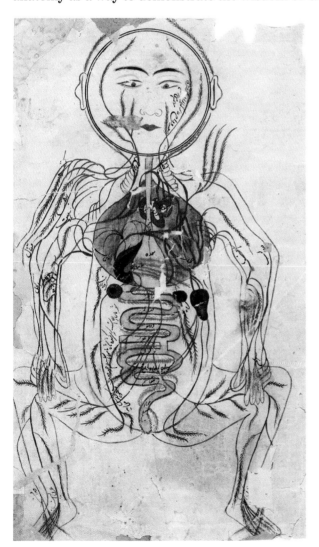

Fig. 31: Mansur, Human nervous system in *Tashrih al-Badan* (Anatomy of the human body), fourteenth to fifteenth century.

have seen circumstantial proof of human dissections in Ibn Nafis's writings, particularly in his suggestion that the heart itself is nourished by blood in the coronary vessels (a very advanced notion for the time).[28] Others have pointed to the anatomic plates in Mansur's work (and similar early Latin illustrations) that show the body face down, with hyperextended head and palms facing backward, suggesting their position on an autopsy table.[29]

Two events had profound impact on the pursuit of medical knowledge and on medical illustration in particular. The first was the invention of the printing press by Gutenberg in 1439. Whereas Galen's had been mostly an oral tradition, the ability to produce printed material on a wide scale allowed the rapid and reproducible distribution of knowledge. The second and more important event was the publication, in 1543, of Andreas Vesalius's masterpiece, *De Humani Corporis Fabrica* (The fabric of the human body). For the first time since Galen's era, someone was able to challenge medical dogma by direct experimentation in the form of thorough and methodical dissection of the human body.

De Humani Corporis Fabrica

Much has been said about the fact that the dissection of human cadavers was prohibited in earlier civilizations, but that is an oversimplification. The Ancient Egyptians had a sophisticated relationship with death and were masters at immortalizing their rulers. However, they were less interested in the body's contents than in the preservation of its shell in as intact a form as possible. Typically, small incisions would be made in the left lower abdomen, through which the internal organs would be removed and preserved separately in canopic jars. Detailed methods of embalming have been amply documented in hieroglyphs, and the end result is visible today in the many museums that exhibit these mummies.

Dissections were practiced in other ancient civilizations, including Greece and the Roman Empire, although human autopsies were outlawed,[30] requiring physicians such as Galen to learn from animal dissections. Andreas Vesalius is generally credited with the first detailed description of the human anatomy, based on painstaking dissections. The seven-volume work is remarkable in its accuracy, and pointedly refutes some of the earlier teachings, all but mentioning Galen by name. The description of the uterus, for example, compares it with the "non-pregnant uterus of the dog" (Fig. 32) with its two uterine horns (unlike the primate organ, which consists of a single cavity). It is hard not to see this as a direct attack on Galen's animal dissections, and in particular the extrapolations of canine anatomy.[31]

As remarkable as Vesalius's work is, he was not the first physician to perform dissections. Autopsies were uncommon in the thirteenth and

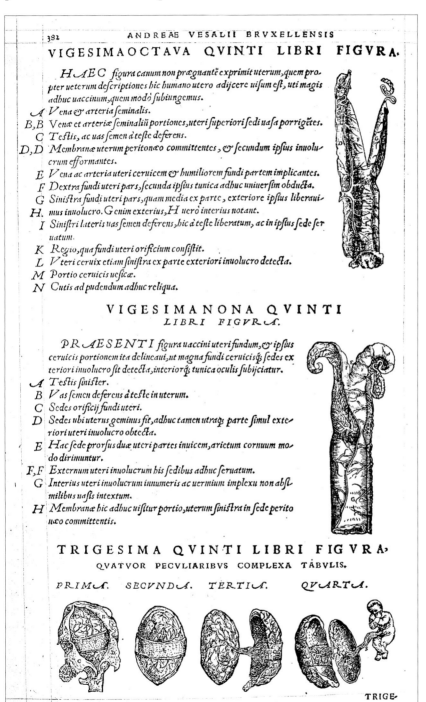

Fig. 32: Andreas Vesalius, Comparative anatomy of the canine (*top*) and human (*bottom*) uterus, in *De Humani Corporis Fabrica* (Of the fabric of the human body), 1543, fifth book, a jab at Galen's teachings about human anatomy that were derived from animal dissections. (Wellcome Images, licensed under CC BY 4.0.)

fourteenth centuries but not unheard of—and sometimes sanctioned by the Catholic Church. In the case of holy figures, an autopsy was a way to understand what made them extraordinary. Two notable examples are cited by Katherine Park in *Secrets of Women*:[32] Margherita of Città di Castello (1320) and Abbess Chiara of Montefalco (1308) were both dissected after death to prove that they were different from the rest of us. The supposed finding of an image of a cross in the Abbess Chiara's heart confirmed her sanctity. In fact, autopsies of women were more common than those of men in an attempt to understand the secrets of pregnancy and childbirth. A well-documented case was that of Fiammetta Admimari, who died in 1477 while giving birth. The autopsy was performed to try and understand what happened. In rare cases, a child could be saved from the womb of a dying mother. This form of cesarean section preceded the first successful cases by several centuries. Here, the goal was not to save the mother.

Naturally, very few individuals could afford to have their bodies dissected after death: autopsies were performed by physicians, often in the home of the deceased, and were a privilege of the rich. Thus, while Judeo-Christian and Islamic mores officially opposed human dissections, there was clearly some wiggle room. This loosening of the laws paved the way for anatomists like Vesalius to further their quest for medical knowledge. While the church clearly restricted the practice of autopsies to physicians (and the occasional religious inquiry), Leonardo da Vinci—famously not a medical doctor—is said to have received special dispensation from the church to do his own dissections. Decades before *De Humani Corporis Fabrica,* he left us numerous sketches of skeletal and muscular anatomy. He even produced now famous drawings of the human fetus in utero (Fig. 33), continuing the fascination people had—and still have—with the hidden anatomy of pregnancy.

Andreas Vesalius is the most famous anatomist of the sixteenth century, but he was actually not the first physician to publish an illustrated atlas of human anatomy. That honor may go to Jacopo Berengario da Carpi, who, in 1522 (two decades before Vesalius) published his *Isagoge Breves Perlucide ac Uberime, in Anatomiam Humani Corporis* (A concise, clear and constructive introduction to the anatomy of the human body), an anatomy textbook containing images of the brain and other illustrations of human dissection.[33] Berengario, a Bolognese surgeon and anatomist with a checkered history, can be seen as a proto-Vesalius, setting the stage for the momentous anatomic discoveries and publications to come, including his repudiation of some of Galen's teachings.

What really sets Vesalius apart are the incredibly detailed and intricate illustrations of his dissections. Herein lies the genius of Vesalius:

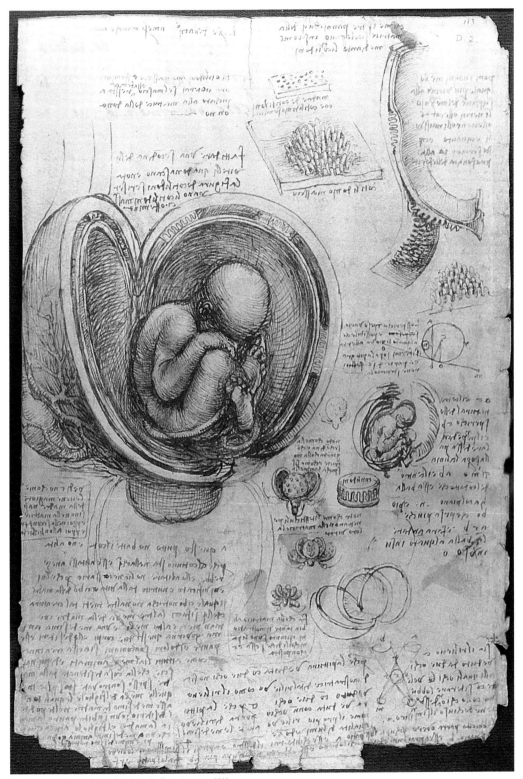

Fig. 33: Leonardo da Vinci, sketches of a fetus in utero, 1511.

his association with artists like Jan Steven Van Calcar, a painter and engraver of the Titian school, thanks to whom this seminal treatise gained notoriety and longevity. This, then, can be considered one of the first deliberate associations between a medical researcher and an illustrator, the beginning of a long tradition that continues to this day. (Van Calcar was likely not the only artist associated with Vesalius's work, and the true provenance of each plate continues to be a matter of debate.[34])

From Hired Hand to Collaborator

Medical illustrators became indispensable for the dissemination of new medical knowledge. As Western society emerged from the Dark Ages, everything about the human body remained to be discovered. Most of the names that are still associated with anatomic structures— the fallopian tubes (after Gabriele Fallopio), the Spiegelian line or linea semilunaris (Adriaan Spiegel), Scarpa's fascia, Glisson's capsule, Cloquet's lymph node, the ampulla of Vater—are named after anatomists who themselves published medical treatises,[35] many of them illustrated with woodcuts or copper plates by famous artists of the day. Spiegel's books were illustrated by Odoardo Fialetti; Charles Etienne's 1545 *De Dissectione Partium Corporis Humani* (The partial dissection of the human body) by Etienne de la Rivière; William Smellie's atlases of midwifery by Peter Camper. Govert Bidloo, a Dutch anatomist and physician, had his *Ontleding des Menschelijken Lichaams* (Dissection of the human body) illustrated by Gerard de Lairesse, a famous painter and contemporary of Rembrandt. In one of the many connections between doctors, diseases, and artists, de Lairesse himself may have suffered from a condition that came to light thanks to a portrait of him by Rembrandt (see chapter 2).

The association between scientist and artist goes back centuries, but a true collaboration between the two professions grew more slowly. Van Calcar has been linked to Vesalius's *De Humani Corporis Fabrica,* but other artists who collaborated with him remained anonymous.[36] Even famous painters like Gerard de Lairesse, who illustrated Bidloo's atlas, were more artists for hire than true partners. Bernhard Siegfried Albinus and Jan Wandelaar, however, are usually mentioned together.[37] The monumental *Tabulae Sceleti et Musculorum Corporis Humani* (Atlas of the skeleton and the muscles of the human body), published in 1747, was the result of a true collaboration between Albinus, a German professor of anatomy at the University of Leiden, and Jan Wandelaar, Dutch painter and engraver. Each man possessed unique and complementary skills and, perhaps not coincidentally, their respective masters had collaborated on similar projects: Albinus's teachers included Bidloo, while Wandelaar's included de Lairesse.

Not merely faithful reproductions of anatomic dissections, Wandelaar's plates were didactic works that extrapolated from a collection of different bodies. He and Albinus created formulas to adapt musculatures and skeletons of different sizes to obtain accurate representations of muscle origins and insertions.[38] The result was one of the most revered works on human anatomy of its time. Although Albinus did not give Wandelaar full credit for his contributions at the time, he did marvel at Wandelaar's preparatory sketches and remarked that artists were astonished that Wandelaar could have made such elaborate engravings from these sketches.[39] In fact, this is seen as one of the strengths of the *Tabulae*'s illustrations: that Jan Wandelaar was not only a great draftsman but a skilled engraver, who produced his own copper plates. The results are images rich with nuances, halftones, and grisaille, giving them a remarkable sense of volume closer to sculptures than to Vesalius's woodcuts (Fig. 34).

Albinus and Wandelaar may have sought to describe the normal, generic anatomy of the human body, but by the middle of the eighteenth century, physicians were running out of anatomic structures to discover. Illustration of normal human anatomy, pioneered by the likes of Vesalius, Spiegel, Fallopio, and Glisson, was naturally followed by the visualization of disease. Before the modern era of medical and surgical therapy, pathological descriptions were skewed toward the monstrous and the grotesque. In the seventeenth century, anatomists and physicians would offer these "Observationes" (essentially, case reports) in dedicated museums or through broadsheet reproductions. One of the earliest and most famous museums was created by Dr. Frederik Ruysch, praelector in anatomy for the Guild of Surgeons in Amsterdam (immortalized in at least two classic paintings; see the introduction). His dioramas, created with the help of his daughter (and famed painter) Rachel Ruysch, ran the gamut from still lives with embalmed or wax-injected body parts amid feathers, jewelry, or shells, to infant or fetal skeletons displayed in naturalistic poses. These elaborate tableaux were often immortalized with exquisitely detailed copper engravings and woodcuts.

The goal of these images of disease was primarily to shock rather than to offer a taxonomy of maladies. In fact, we find more about representations of disease in religious or artistic contexts than in medical treatises of that era.[40] From skin conditions to venereal diseases, classical art is replete with the depiction of common medical conditions.

Even when the intent was scientific pursuit, academic physicians like John Hunter (1728–93) were attracted mostly by the unusual and the grotesque. Hunter's chance encounter with Charles Byrne, the "Irish giant," is one great example (see chapter 3).

John Hunter is considered a pioneer of modern surgery and a much sought-after clinician. He and his older brother William also led popular autopsy sessions for the educated public in London. In

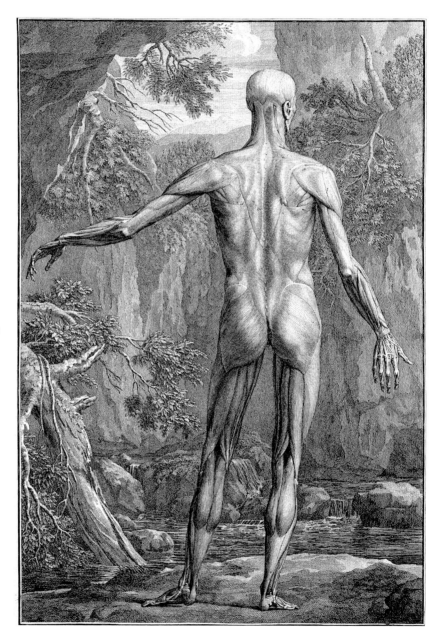

Fig. 34: Bernhard Siegfried Albinus and Jan Wandelaar, *Tabulae Sceleti et Musculorum Corporis Humani* (Plates of the skeleton and the muscles of the human body), table V, 1749. Note the rich monochrome palette of this copper engraving, a significant improvement over the black-and-white woodcuts of Vesalius's *De Humani Corporis Fabrica* (Figs. 2 and 32). (Courtesy of the National Library of Medicine.)

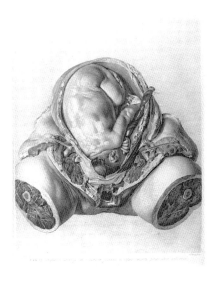
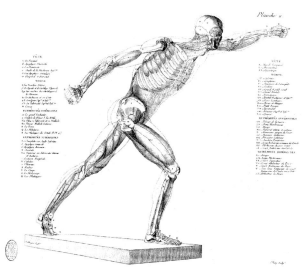

addition to these highly attended classes, William Hunter published several treatises on human anatomy with an emphasis—again—on pregnancy and childbirth. These were lavishly illustrated by Jan van Rymsdyk, a famous medical illustrator and engraver from the Netherlands (Fig. 35).

The brothers Hunter were brilliant anatomists but had to rely on van Rymsdyk's talents to illustrate their work. A few decades later, Jean-Galbert Salvage, a physician and surgeon educated at the venerable medical school of Montpellier, France, wanted to have it all. He set out to combine his knowledge of anatomy, his experience as a military surgeon, and his artistic abilities into the definitive atlas of anatomy. His work is a perfect example of the blurred lines between art, medicine, and scientific illustration (Fig. 36). Two of the plates for his *Anatomie du Gladiateur Combatant* (Anatomy of the fighting gladiator) were exhibited at the 1804 Salon of the Académie des Beaux-Arts of Paris, the most prestigious annual art exhibition in Europe for more than two centuries (and the site of several famous "scandals" that ushered in impressionism and other nonclassical art movements—see chapter 3.)[41]

Salvage's atlas did not become a world classic as he had hoped. Another physician-artist did manage to achieve that goal: Henry Vandyke Carter, who graduated with a degree in medicine from the University of London in 1857, had already been working as a freelance artist for the *Lancet* when he was approached by Henry Gray, professor of anatomy at St. George's Hospital in London, to illustrate a comprehensive textbook of human anatomy. *Anatomy, Descriptive and Surgical* was first

Fig. 35: William Hunter, table XX, from *The Anatomy of the Human Gravid Uterus Exhibited in Figures*, 1774. Illustration by Jan van Rymsdyk.

Fig. 36: Jean-Galbert Salvage, *Anatomie du Gladiateur Combattant* (Anatomy of the fighting gladiator), plate 10, 1812. (Wellcome Images, licensed under CC BY 4.0.)

published in 1858 and is still one of the most widely known and used atlases in the world (Fig. 37). The latest edition, published in 2020 and edited by Dr. Susan Standring, is its forty-second. Although Henry Vandyke Carter's medical illustrations achieved the notoriety that Dr. Salvage had craved, Carter himself did not reap its benefits. He was paid minimally for the work and had to fight to obtain due credit. Henry Vandyke Carter is now mostly remembered for his work in tropical medicine and his discovery of a spirochete,[42] while the seminal work he made famous is simply called *Gray's Anatomy*.

While the seventeenth and eighteenth centuries had been marked by rapid discoveries in human anatomy, medical advances were scarce. Experimental pharmacology was nonexistent, and the good outcome of most surgical interventions was threatened by a lack of understand-

Fig. 37: Henry Vandyke Carter, Veins of the head and neck, in Henry Gray, *Anatomy, Descriptive and Surgical* (*Gray's Anatomy*), 11th ed., 1887.

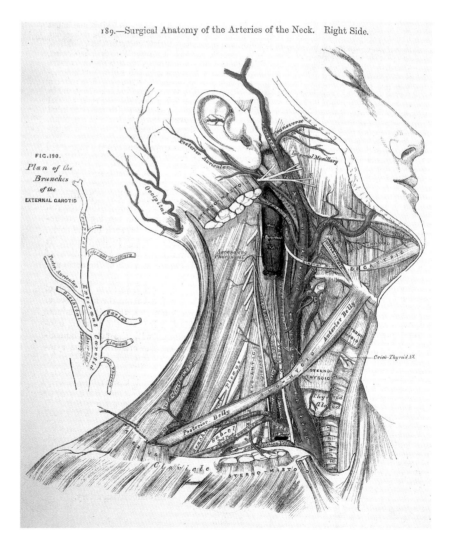

ing of infections, the inability to control bleeding, and the scarcity of adequate instrumentation.

There were exceptions, of course. Some enlightened scientists attempted to deduce physiologic principles from their observations and applied those in the treatment of an increasing number of conditions. One of the most notorious examples is John Hunter's observations regarding the popliteal aneurysm, a professional hazard of carriage coach drivers.[43] As the hard benches and lack of suspension would cause repetitive trauma to the back of the thigh, just above the knee, the wall of the underlying popliteal artery would weaken and bulge out. The aneurysm would gradually increase in size and invariably rupture, either causing gangrene of the lower leg by interrupting its blood supply or leading to exsanguination. Either way, the patient would eventually die unless the leg could be amputated before the rupture of the aneurysm—a daunting prospect that would also rob him of his income, if he could no longer work. John Hunter used his anatomic knowledge (the popliteal artery emerges through a sharp-edged hole in the fascia as it travels behind the knee) to understand how the aneurysm developed, and deduced that ligature of the artery just above it could save the patient's limb. This opening in the fascia is now known as Hunter's canal.

Surgery did not become a true specialty until a century later, thanks in great part to the discovery of asepsis (by the likes of Louis Pasteur and Joseph Lister) and the introduction of anesthesia (usually credited to dentist William Morton in 1846). As a result, operations, while still often dangerous, became at least feasible. Whereas two centuries before, medical atlases focused on anatomy, newer textbooks were about therapies. The apprenticeship model of teaching medicine and surgery was popular enough—you would absorb knowledge by observing the master, and students would travel great distances to learn from the best—and that didactic model is still in use today, albeit to a much lesser extent. But the best way to reach larger audiences was through printed material, and the most effective method to teach the finer points and perils of new operations was through medical illustration.

A perfect example of the transition between classic anatomic plates and practical medical textbooks is the *Traité Complet de l'Anatomie de l'Homme* (Complete treatise of human anatomy), the masterwork of Jean-Baptiste Bourgery and Nicholas Jacob, published in installments between 1831 and 1840. As Jean-Marie Le Minor remarks in the introduction to an expanded 2012 edition based on the original atlas, Bourgery and Jacob's work "cover[s] descriptive anatomy, surgical anatomy and techniques (exploring in detail nearly all the major operations that were performed during the first half of the 19th century)."[44] The figures of the initial edition were in black and white, printed using the technique of lithography that was invented only a few decades earlier. The second edition contained many color lithographs (Fig. 38) that were remarkable for their lifelike, photographic qualities, a testament to the converging movements in art and medicine that ushered in the modern era of medical illustration.[45] The "Bourgery & Jacob" is also one of the first examples of physician and illustrator getting equal billing—the start of true collaboration.

When the Johns Hopkins University in Baltimore created its medical school, they recruited four famous physicians: William Halsted, already a renowned surgeon; William Osler, the illustrious internist from McGill University in Montreal; the gynecologist Howard Kelly; and the pathologist William Welch. In 1888, when Kelly started to write his landmark textbooks on gynecological surgery, he needed them to be illustrated. Just like their colleagues from Italy, the Netherlands, and France centuries earlier, Kelly and Halsted recruited an artist, the German painter Max Brödel, convincing him to leave Leipzig for

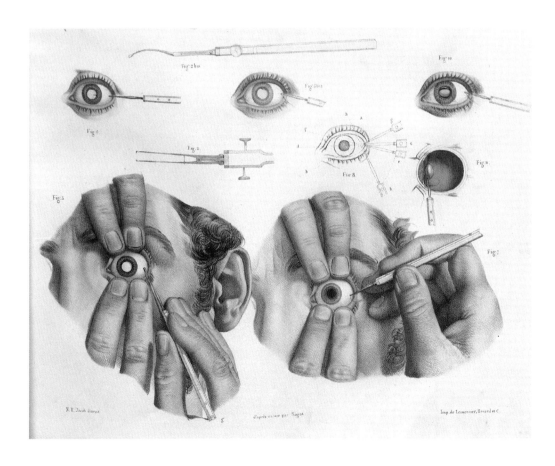

Baltimore. Brödel was not only a gifted artist, but he developed newer techniques to best serve the needs of a surgical atlas—black-and-white pen drawings and grayscale illustrations using carbon dust, an improvement on charcoal that produced crisp, highly contrasted images that were superbly detailed and ideal for printed reproduction (Fig. 39). Howard Kelly's textbooks were successful in large part thanks to the many illustrations of the often-daring surgical procedures as these images were so much more useful than text alone to teach generations of gynecologists and surgeons. Brödel's success was such that he became known as the "Fifth Doctor" at Johns Hopkins Hospital. In 1911,

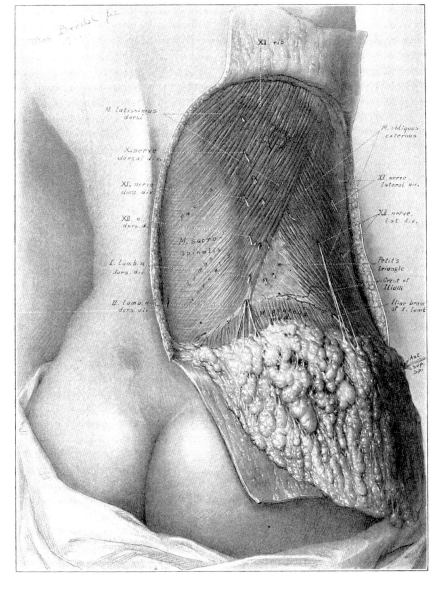

Fig. 39: Max Brödel, Carbon dust technique of medical illustration, in Howard A. Kelly, *Diseases of the Kidneys, Ureters and Bladder*, 1922.

thanks to a large grant from Henry Walters, a Baltimore financier and philanthropist, Max Brödel was able to head his own full-fledged department of medical illustration at Hopkins—the Department of Art as applied to Medicine.[46] This was the very first school of medical illustration in North America, and many of its students went on to become masters and innovators in medical illustration throughout the continent and the world. Max Brödel is considered one of the fathers of this profession, and Johns Hopkins the birthplace of modern medical illustration in North America.[47]

Chapter 2

The Accidental Medical Illustrator

The Artist as Observer

Medical illustration is the marriage between art and medicine with the intent to enhance communication. There is a lot of medicine in art—depictions of diseases, syndromes, and other ailments in paintings and sculptures throughout history. Classic paintings may portray royalty (Fig. 40) and nobility (often because these were the people who paid artists for their work), depict religious or mythological events (Fig. 41), or bear witness to more mundane scenes of daily lives. Regardless of the subject, all great masterpieces are feats of observation, and they can reveal so much to the attentive eye. In their detailed reproduction of the human body, they also divulge basic medical information.

Unbeknown to the casual viewer, many diseases and conditions can be found in these works of art, from dwarfism (Fig. 40) to Down syndrome (Fig. 41),[1] either because artists faithfully reproduced the features of their subjects, or because they sought to insert familiar features into unrelated compositions. Sometimes these hidden treasures generate the satisfaction of finding Easter eggs—the pleasure of knowing something others don't know, or discovering a feature that was hiding in plain sight for centuries. Of course, the true explanation behind these "pearls" is often the result of speculation, as the motivation of artists and the exact nature of their compositions are mostly lost. In some cases, speculations border on conspiracy theories, as when famous artists are believed by some to have hidden elaborate messages in their works out of fear of persecution. The Sistine Chapel

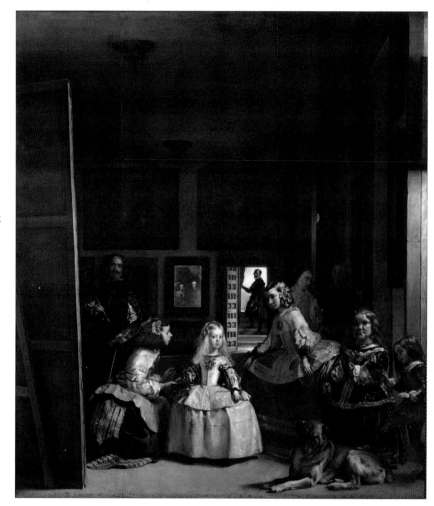

Fig. 40: Diego Velazquez, *Las Meninas* (The maids of honor), 1656. Members of the royal Spanish court, including the infanta Margaret Theresa (center), her ladies-in-waiting, and the German dwarf Maria Barbola (*right*), 1656. The painter (*left*) is finishing the portrait of King Philip IV and his wife, whom we see reflected in the mirror in the back, just above the infanta's head.

frescoes, for example, are said to hold proof that Michelangelo had an advanced knowledge of human anatomy, acquired through many human dissections. The iconic image of God, in the *Creation of Adam,* is surrounded by angels whose heads are strangely clustered and enveloped by a bizarrely draped red cloak. Frank Meshberger first advanced the theory (later expanded by Ian Suk, a professor of medical illustration, and Rafael Tamargo, a neurosurgeon) that Michelangelo Buonarotti was not only an artistic genius but also a master anatomist.[2] The draping and the group of angels surrounding God bear an uncanny resemblance to the human brain, complete with brainstem and medulla (Fig. 42). Suk and Tamargo point to other examples of anatomic structures hidden in the frescoes' design, such as the optic chasm, the kidney, and a ventral view of the brainstem in the *Separation of Light from Darkness* panel.[3] We will, of course, never know

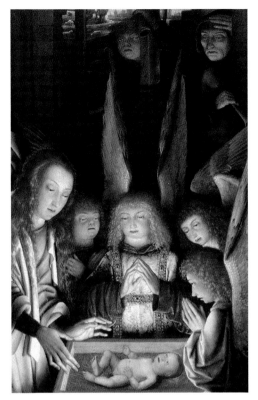

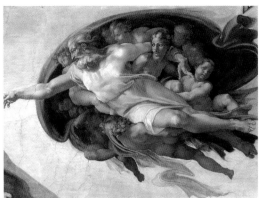

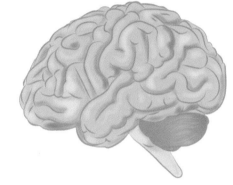

Fig. 41: Student of Jan Joest, *Adoration of the Christ Child* (detail), circa 1550. Although the subject is religious and refers to the birth of Christ, the execution of this Flemish masterpiece reflects fashion, customs, and aspects of daily life in the era of the painter, including two characters with clear features of Down syndrome (the angel immediately to the right of the Virgin Mary and the peasant above him).

Fig. 42: Michelangelo Buonarotti, *The Creation of Adam,* ceiling, Sistine Chapel (detail). Ian Suk and Rafael Tamargo have argued that the figure of God, surrounded by angels and a peculiar draping, is a not-so-subtle description of the human brain. (*Bottom image:* Injurymap, licensed under CC BY 4.0.)

Michelangelo's true intentions or the extent of his anatomic knowledge. There are other clues that he knew "a little too much" about human anatomy, however, such as the existence of the sartorius muscle in the thigh, a structure that is not visible externally, and would have been encountered only through dissections. If so, he would not likely have wanted to flaunt his anatomic expertise when the church was strongly opposed to nonmedical autopsies. (How do we know he knew about the sartorius? Because he famously added its impression in paintings and sculptures, one of several Michelangelo idiosyncrasies that have helped authenticate his work.[4])

There is no denying the close relationship between art, medical science, and medical illustration. And it is not always clear who copied whom, as in the example of the flayed man (Fig. 43): Vesalius, in his 1543

De Humani Corporis Fabrica, describes the superficial musculature in a plate in which the skin and subcutaneous tissues of the body have been removed, a figure that is known in nonmedical artistic circles as an *écorché* (French for *flayed*). Ecorché paintings and sculptures became popular in the Renaissance—da Vinci produced some of the most famous ones—and have been a staple of art school exercises since. Only a few years before Vesalius's publication, Michelangelo depicted St.

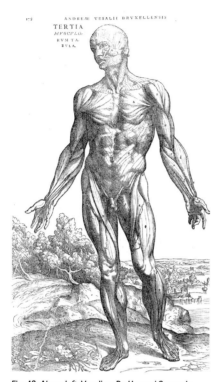

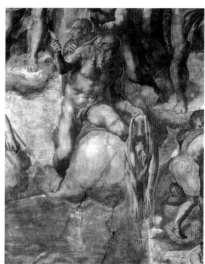

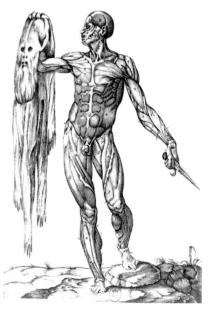

Fig. 43: *Above left:* Vesalius, *De Humani Corporis Fabrica* (Of the fabric of the human body), 1543, second book: Superficial musculature, exposed after removing the skin (flaying). Above *right:* Michelangelo Buonarotti, *The Last Judgement,* Sistine Chapel, 1536–41 (detail): St. Bartholomew holding the two attributes of his martyrdom: the flaying knife and his entire body's skin. *Right:* Gaspar Becerra, in Juan Valverde de Hamusco, *Historia de la Composición del Cuerpo Humano* (History of the composition of the human body), circa 1520–70. The illustration, sometimes incorrectly attributed to Vesalius, appears to be inspired by Vesalius's work as well as that of Michelangelo.

Bartholomew holding his own skin and a skinning knife, symbolizing his martyrdom; this is not to say that Vesalius copied Michelangelo, but Becerra's anatomic treatise seems to have borrowed from both: the anatomic model shows off his muscles *and* his discarded skin.

The Physician as Observer

Classic art is a reflection of its time, whether in the depiction of fashion, scenery, architecture, or occupations. It also holds a treasure trove of medical information, some of which has been very well documented and corroborated. Looking for medical clues in the work of old masters can be rewarding at multiple levels. There is the satisfaction of detecting well-known conditions such as Down syndrome, giving us somewhat of a connection with our ancestors. It confirms that things haven't changed that much after all. It teaches us about the greater context of medicine in society, like the acceptance (and sometimes reverence) of those who are different than us, such as people with dwarfism. Beyond the treasure-hunt qualities of this exercise, looking for explanations or backstories behind classic paintings can also be beneficial to medical students, trainees, and practicing physicians.[5] Trying to understand a character's problems, even if they are fictive, can enhance our sense of compassion and empathy—and certainly hone our observational skills. A growing number of medical schools now offer art appreciation courses, and team up with museum curators to analyze great works of art with students and doctors-in-training—the better to bring humanism (back) to medicine.[6] In the midst of the most revolutionary era in science and technology, there is a clear movement to return to the importance of the doctor-patient relationship, the one-on-one bond of trust between human beings free of computers, batteries of tests, and—gasp—electronic health records that all conspire to overtake our lives, Terminator-style. What is the difference, after all, between the elaborate history-taking and examination of a patient and the scrutiny of a detailed painting, looking for body-language hints behind the expressions and poses of the characters? Notice the clothes each person is wearing? Accessories and attributes of social standing? Scars on their hands or faces? Can these be clues to their occupation and perhaps to their ailment? Most importantly, the time it takes to truly look at a painting is more than a metaphor for the time doctors need to reclaim to really listen, observe, and relate to their patients, oblivious to other activities and obligations that are all competing for our attention in our busy schedule.[7]

There is little doubt that art can be enriching to physicians, possibly teaching them better observational skills and bedside manners. Furthermore, medicine is amply represented in classic art. Still, the depiction of medical conditions or surgical practices in masterworks does not make them medical illustrations. What is lacking is a clear didactic purpose, an image whose goal is to educate, clarify, or instruct in the clearest possible way; whether it can also be considered artistic is a secondary benefit. That does not mean, however, that classic art cannot be didactic as well, either as a tool to bring humanism to medicine, or as a direct representation of disease that we cannot obtain any other way. Many paintings may not have started as medical illustrations, but they can be considered as such after the fact as they offer information that cannot be obtained by any other means.

Documenting Defunct Diseases

When Diego Velazquez painted dwarfs at the king's court, he was merely reflecting life in seventeenth-century Spain. The condition was not yet known as achondroplasia, and its genetic background had not been unraveled, but the features of the condition are as recognizable today as they were in Velazquez's lifetime. Other diseases would have been much more prevalent centuries ago, however, and virtually unknown today. Unhygienic living conditions and limited medical knowledge were responsible for diseases that either don't exist anymore or can now be treated before they develop full-blown symptoms. (Conversely, certain medical conditions are "modern" and a direct consequence of progress—from radiation-induced cancers to motor vehicle injuries.)

Among the "forgotten" medical conditions are many infectious diseases. For millennia, smallpox was prevalent in most of the world. It is estimated that in eighteenth-century Europe, smallpox was responsible for four hundred thousand deaths each year, and was the leading cause of blindness.[8] A prime example of effective healthcare policy that is more relevant than ever today, the elimination of this once-feared infectious disease is intimately linked to the development of vaccination. In 1980, the World Health Organization officially declared smallpox eradicated.[9] Few people today have ever seen the sequelae of smallpox, and fewer still would recognize an acute presentation of the disease. In 1626, sixteen-year-old Ferdinando II de Medici was immortalized by Justus Sustermans, the family portrait painter, on the seventh and ninth days after he contracted smallpox (Fig. 44). The fact that he was previously healthy (as we know from earlier portraits),

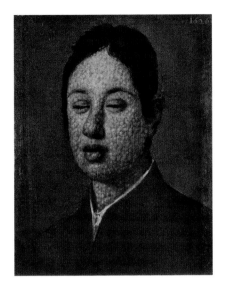
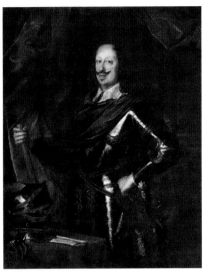

Fig. 44: Justus Sustermans, Portraits of Ferdinando II de Medici. *Left:* Nine days after the onset of smallpox, 1626. The innumerable papules across the entire face and neck are all in the same stage; a similar portrait, two days earlier, showed blotchy erythema, the prodrome of the full syndrome. *Right:* Ferdinando II as Grand Duke of Tuscany, 1632-54. The disease has apparently left no sequelae, a rare occurrence for a condition that caused significant scarring and often led to blindness.

the sudden and simultaneous appearance of erythematous blotches over the entire body (seen in the first of the two portraits), and the synchronous evolution to typical fluid-filled papules two days later leave little doubt as to the cause of this condition.[10] Later portraits of Ferdinando II show that he was lucky enough to recover without any significant scars or sequelae. It is obvious that Sustermans's intentions were to document, not to teach. Today, however, his paintings vividly illustrate a disease that almost no contemporary doctors have seen in their lifetime. The last naturally occurring outbreak happened in the mid-1970s, although the virus persisted in numerous laboratories around the world for decades after that. Today, all laboratory stocks of smallpox should have been destroyed, but some scientists argue that tightly controlled preservation of some samples may be beneficial to the development of future vaccines. As recent events have shown, the risk that a laboratory leak could lead to an outbreak, or even a pandemic, is no longer a farfetched movie scenario—it is being debated with renewed urgency today.[11] Whether accidental or intentional, resurgence of smallpox remains a theoretical threat, and the pockmarked face of Ferdinando de Medici, as documented chronologically by the family artist, can be seen as a timeless diagnostic tool.

Another often fulminant disease that is now almost unheard of is ergotism, an infection with the fungus *Claviceps purpura*, which is typically found in rotting rye and other cereals. The toxins released by the fungus, including ergotamine, are alkaloids with strong vasoconstrictive and neurotoxic properties, leading to many of the symptoms of the disease. These include seizures, gangrene of extremities, nausea and

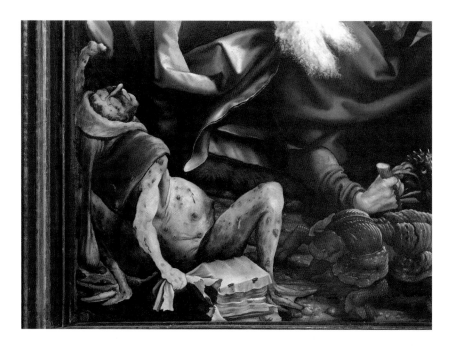

Fig. 45: Matthias Grünewald, *The Temptation of Saint Anthony* (detail), 1512-16. The agonizing peasant in the foreground is covered in pustules and sores and has severe abdominal distension, signs interpreted by some as ergotism, also known as St. Anthony's fire.

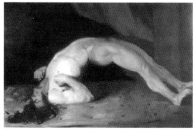

Fig. 46: Charles Bell, Tetanus: *Opisthotonus*, 1844.

vomiting, and other gastrointestinal manifestations. (Ergotamine has been used to treat migraine because of its cerebrovascular properties; a synthetic ergot alkaloid, methylergometrine, is a staple of obstetric medicine, and is used after delivery to effect hemostasis by vasoconstriction as the placenta separates from the uterus.) The German painter Matthias Grünewald, a contemporary of Albrecht Dürer, was commissioned to paint the altarpiece by the monks of the monastery of St. Anthony in Isenheim (near Colmar, France). The Antonine monks were renowned for caring for sufferers of the plague and ergotism, which is also called St. Anthony's fire. The panel of the triptych that represents *The Temptation of Saint Anthony* shows several characters afflicted by a skin condition classically identified as ergotism (Fig. 45).[12]

In early nineteenth-century Edinburgh, Dr. Charles Bell blurred the lines between medicine, medical illustration, and art. A great artist himself, he depicted many syndromes he treated in vivid detail to serve as examples for his students.[13] One of these is tetanus, the spastic

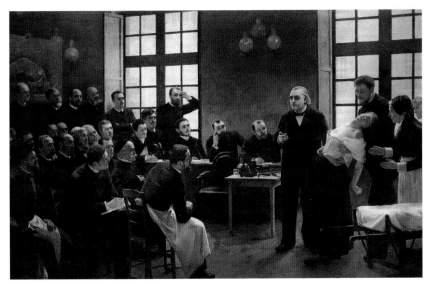

paralysis seen in late stages of untreated infections with *Clostridium tetani* (Fig. 46). That these drawings have survived is priceless as many of the diseases they depict, like tetanus and poliomyelitis, have been all but eradicated.[14]

The arched back and spine in Bell's illustration resemble a condition depicted in another famous painting: *A Clinical Lesson at the Salpêtrière* (Fig. 47). In this case, the condition (epilepsy) is still very much prevalent today, but its etiology has been cleared up. The scene shows Dr. Jean-Martin Charcot and a patient who has seemingly fainted, possibly a manifestation of hysteria (epilepsy), a condition that was then believed to be typical for women. On the far wall, toward the top left of the painting, is a large illustration of another phase of the condition, the *arc de cercle* or arching, like that seen with tetany—an illustration by Paul Richer, anatomist, medical illustrator, and assistant to Dr. Charcot (Fig. 48). Paul Richer's other claim to fame is his 1889 *Artistic Anatomy,* one of the most important works on human external anatomy and an alleged source of reference for many contemporary French painters, such as Renoir and Degas.[15] The original French edition is now a rare collector's item, but an English translation, first published in 1971, is still available.

The fact that many contagious diseases have now nearly disappeared—from tetanus and diphtheria to whooping cough and poliomyelitis—owes everything to smallpox, the primordial vaccination story: from its etymologic origin (*vaccine* refers to *vacca*, Latin for *cow*, as in cowpox) to its worldwide eradication in 1980. The folk story of Edward Jenner, who noted that milkmaids who had had cowpox

Fig. 48: Paul Richer, *Arc de cercle* (arching) phase of a hysterical attack, in Paul Richer, *Etudes Cliniques de l'Hystéro-Epilepsie* (Clinical studies on hystero-epilepsy), 1884.

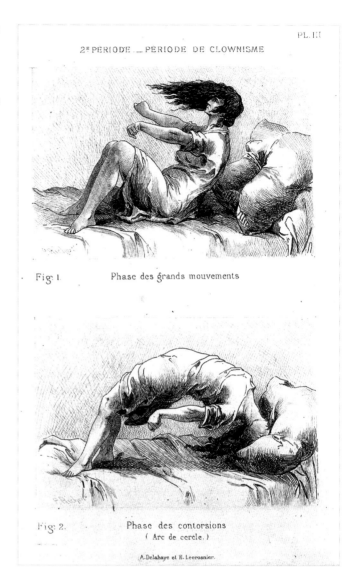

never suffered from smallpox or its disfiguring effects, is well known and amply depicted in art (Fig. 49).[16] What is remarkable is that the history of immunization against viruses predates the discovery of the germ theory by almost a century. It would take the likes of Oliver Wendell Holmes, Ignaz Semmelweis, Louis Pasteur, who all recognized that puerperal fever was a contagion; Robert Koch, who identified the microorganisms responsible for many diseases; and Joseph Lister, who introduced antiseptic practices, to usher in the modern era of infectiology.

As with the example of hysteria and epilepsy, many of the diseases that are still around today are much better understood. Early pre-

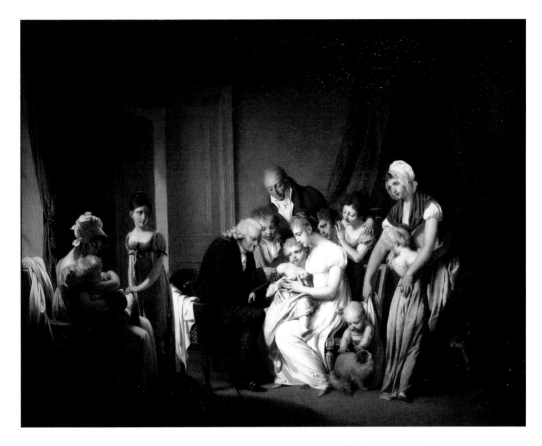

Fig. 49: Louis Boilly,
*La Vaccine ou Le
Préjugé Vaincu* (The
vaccine or prejudice
defeated), 1807.

ventive measures can be taken to avoid progression of a disease, and behavior can be modified to avoid the risk altogether. This is especially true for diseases that can be passed on from a pregnant mother to her unborn child, so-called vertical transmission. A prime example is congenital syphilis, and it is depicted in a harrowing way by Edvard Munch's *The Inheritance,* his 1899 painting of a mother grieving over her dying infant (Fig. 50).[17]

Syphilis had first been described by Girolamo Fracastroro,[18] a Veronese physician whose portrait by Titian hangs in London's National Gallery. (Titian is indirectly related to medical illustration: it was one of his students, Jan Steven Van Calcar, who illustrated Vesalius's seminal *De Humani Corporis Fabrica* in 1543.) By the time Munch painted *The Inheritance,* the disease had been well studied, and its cause was soon to be identified (the *Treponema pallidum* bacteria). In previous centuries, venereal diseases were not distinguishable from one another, and what was known as "great pox" (a major early manifestation of which were the pockmarks that it left) could refer to syphilis (Fig. 51), gonorrhea, or many other sexually transmitted diseases. A well-known representation of these skin lesions can be found in the work of William Hogarth (Fig.

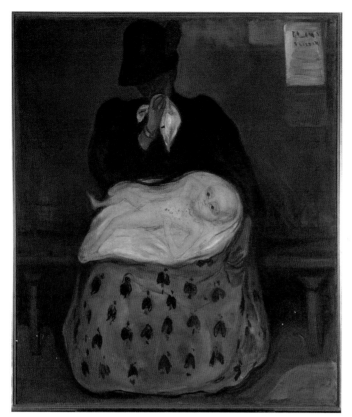
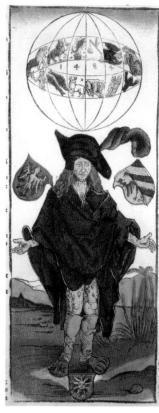

Fig. 50: Edvard Munch, *The Inheritance,* 1889. The newborn child shows signs of congenital syphilis, which will prove fatal.

Fig. 51: Albrecht Dürer, The syphilitic man, in Theodoricus Ulsenius, *Vaticinium in Epidemicam Scabiem* (Prediction of a scabies epidemic), 1496. Note that before the discovery of the pathogens for syphilis and other venereal infections, disease names were often used interchangeably. What is called scabies here is also referred to as *morbus Gallicus* (French disease) or syphilis.

52).[19] (Smallpox, famously not a venereal disease, was so named to differentiate it from great pox.)

While congenital syphilis can be lethal, it does not always have a dismal prognosis. It does, however, have characteristic sequelae that are very rarely seen today. Here, again, classic art may have an accidental role in teaching us the signs and symptoms of long-forgotten diseases. One of the best-known examples of congenital syphilis in art is the portrait of Gerard de Lairesse, a prolific Dutch painter and, later, medical illustrator. De Lairesse was a well-respected artist in Amsterdam in the seventeenth century, the Dutch Golden Age, and is remembered for many baroque works, including painted ceilings in the *herenhuizen* (mansions) of the Amsterdam elite. The opulence of the Netherlands at the time, resulting from the Dutch trade hegemony, is exemplified by works like *Allegory on Concord, Freedom and Security,* a triptic by de Lairesse for then mayor of Amsterdam Andries de Graeff.

Gerard de Lairesse was hired by Govert Bidloo—renowned doctor, anatomist, and the personal physician of William III of Orange-Nassau—to illustrate his treatise on human anatomy, *Ontleding*

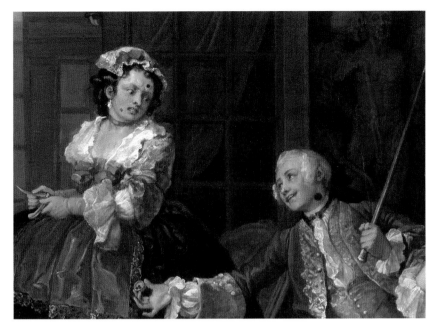

Fig. 52: William Hogarth, *Marriage à la mode 3: The inspection* (details), 1743. Black spots (pox) on face and neck are a manifestation of syphilis.

der Menschelyken Lichaams (Dissection of the human body), another example of a physician-illustrator collaboration in the tradition of Vesalius and Van Calcar.[20] But what is especially interesting in the person of Gerard de Lairesse is his physiognomy. In addition to a number of self-portraits that show him at different stages of adult life, there is a well-known portrait of him by Rembrandt (Fig. 53). It shows a young de Lairesse staring directly at us, with peculiar features that have been interpreted by many as representing the phenotype of congenital syphilis.[21] Typical facial characteristics of late congenital syphilis include a "boyish" appearance, prominent forehead, marked frontal eminences, a long philtrum (the vertical groove between nose and mouth), hypoplasia of the nose bridge that gives the nose an up-turned aspect, prominent lips, and fine grooves at the corners of the mouth. The disease, which is transmitted from an infected mother, has many other features that affect most organ systems, but there is no way, of course, to confirm de Lairesse's diagnosis. It is known that he became blind later in life, and blindness (through involvement of the optic nerves by the disease) is a late manifestation of syphilis, but causality cannot be established. Whether true or not, this iconic painting by Rembrandt is often used as an illustration of congenital syphilis. It is, above all, a useful image of a disease that few clinicians, if any, will ever see in their careers.

Congenital syphilis has been described as the "sins of the mother," since it is transmitted vertically from an infected pregnant woman

Fig. 53: *Right:* Rembrandt van Rijn, *Portrait of Gerard de Lairesse,* 1665–67. Note the upturned nose, long philtrum, wrinkles at the mouth corners, all possible features of congenital syphilis. *Below left:* Typical face of a young man with congenital syphilis, in Byron Bramwell, *Atlas of Clinical Medicine,* 1893, p. 82. (Science History Images/Alamy Stock Photo.)

Below right: Fig. 54: Benjamin Robert Haydon, *John Keats,* 1816. The profile shows some features also seen in fetal alcohol syndrome: small forehead, low nasal bridge, thin upper lip, and flat midface. (Photograph by Arthur Dawson © National Portrait Gallery, London.)

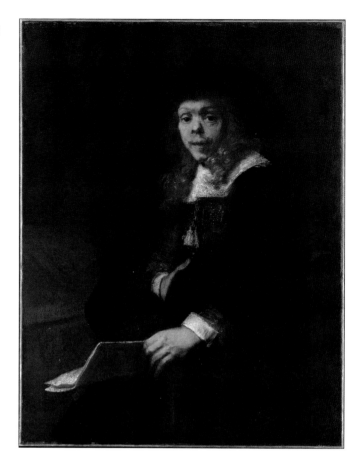

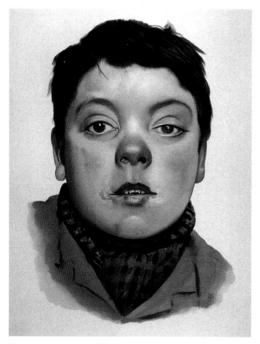

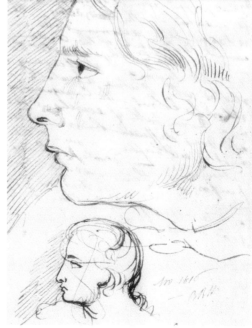

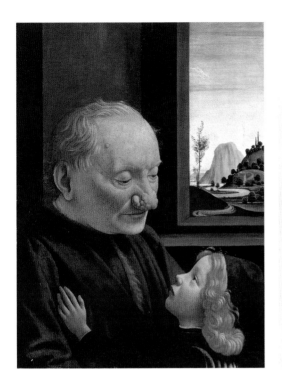
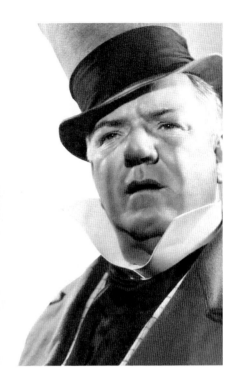

to her unborn child. Throughout history, syphilis and other venereal diseases have been blamed on promiscuity and prostitution, and therefore disproportionately on women. The expression *femme fatale* probably refers to it, as does the poem by John Keats, "La Belle Dame sans Merci" (The merciless lady).[22] In an ironic twist, Keats (whose rumors about contracting syphilis have been debunked[23]) may have been the victim of the sins of his mother—of a different kind. It has been suggested recently that his small forehead, thin upper lip, low nasal bridge (Fig. 54), and hand features were all signs of fetal alcohol syndrome—a result of excessive maternal alcohol intake during pregnancy.[24] While the dangers of alcohol consumption by pregnant women have been known for centuries (observations about its effects were reported during the eighteenth-century gin epidemic in England), the syndrome was recognized as a true entity only in 1973.

Alcoholism remains a public health concern, but some extreme manifestations may be rarely seen today as early intervention is more widespread. The old man in *An Old Man and His Grandson* (Fig. 55) exhibits such an obsolete sign: he has papular rosacea of the nose, or rhinophyma, a common finding with advanced age that is also seen in individuals with alcoholic cirrhosis.[25] This phenomenon became the "red nose" shorthand representation of drunks in caricatures, comic books, and comedies.

Fig. 55: *Left: Domenico Ghirlandaio, An Old Man and His Grandson,* circa 1490. A pronounced form of rosacea that involves raised red papules on the tip of the nose, seen in old age and in cases of alcoholic cirrhosis, is often seen in caricatures and comics (think W. C. Fields, *right*) to indicate that someone is drunk.

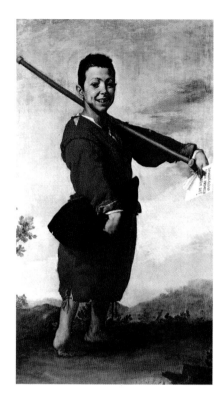

Fig. 56: Jusepe de Ribera, *El Patizambo, o el Pie Varo* (Bowlegs, or the clubfoot), 1642.

Other afflictions that would have been more common centuries ago include clubfoot, a condition that can now be corrected through orthopedic surgery (Fig. 56), and goiter, a disease of the thyroid gland that is often a result of iodine deficiency. So-called endemic goiter was prevalent in noncoastal regions without access to iodine-rich sea salt. Nowadays, table salt is fortified with iodine, and endemic goiter has largely disappeared in developed countries. The most prominent feature of a goiter is a significantly enlarged thyroid gland, visible as a large lump in the anterior neck (Fig. 57). As with many other "medical conditions" in art, we do not know for sure whether the characters depicted in these paintings truly had a goiter, but that condition would have been prevalent enough that a painter's model might have been affected by it. While large goiters are not unknown to endocrinologists and endocrine surgeons today, they are rare enough that most general practitioners may be less familiar with the disease. Recognizing an uncommon condition from a classic painting can be a useful adjunct to its description in a medical textbook.

One condition that was prevalent in specific regions of the world is beta thalassemia. Centuries ago, it was particularly rampant in Southern European countries. Thalassemia is still very much a health problem today, but whereas it is much less prevalent in the Western world, including the Mediterranean basin, it is endemic in Southeast Asia. As our world is becoming increasingly global, North American doctors today are exposed to diseases and conditions that may not have been covered well in medical school. Beta thalassemia is one of these conditions. Because of a genetic defect in one of the two chains of hemoglobin, the oxygen-carrying capacity of red blood cells is impaired, and the body must produce these cells at a much higher rate. Ordinarily, red blood cells are produced in the bone marrow of the long bones, but when demand rises significantly, other bones contribute as well. This is particularly true for the bones of the skull (which are normally flat and contain much less marrow). This medullary overgrowth causes the frontal bone, among others, to expand, a phenomenon called frontal bossing. The unfinished *The Manchester Madonna* by Michelangelo is said to show frontal bossing in the figure of John the Baptist (Fig.

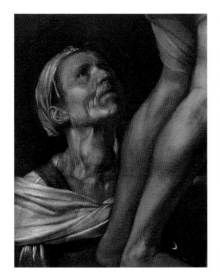

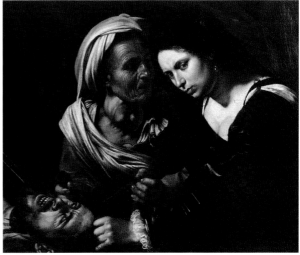

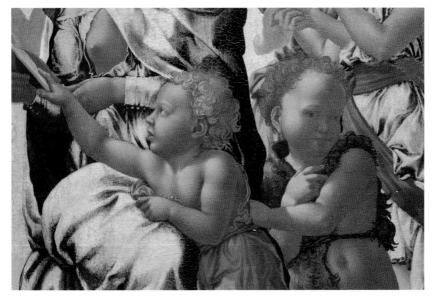

Above: Fig. 57: Goiter or enlarged thyroid gland, seen as a midline swelling of the neck. *Left:* Caravaggio, *The Crucifixion of St. Andrews* (detail), circa 1607. *Right:* Presumed Caravaggio, *Judith Beheading Holofernes* (detail), circa 1606.

Left: Fig. 58: Michelangelo, *The Manchester Madonna,* 1497. While the young Jesus (*left*) has a normally shaped head, John the Baptist (*right,* depicted as usual wearing an animal skin) shows frontal bossing.

58).[26] While nobody suggests that John the Baptist suffered from thalassemia, it is not impossible that Michelangelo (who, after all, lived in a region where the condition was endemic) could have used as model a child with thalassemia. In the painting, the contrast between the normal shape of the young Jesus's head and the prominent forehead of John the Baptist is striking. It becomes a useful didactic tool for a disease manifestation that is not very common today.

Medical illustrations can be pieces of art, but not every piece of art with a medical subject qualifies as a medical illustration. While artists may convey a message, it is not necessarily a didactic one. In some cases, however, a disease is inextricably tied to a work of art. One of the most famous examples is a condition associated with the royal family who ruled most of Europe for hundreds of years. Members of the Habsburg dynasty are found in every European court between the sixteenth and the eighteenth century. The chief phenotypic feature of the Habsburgs was pronounced prognathism (prominent lower jaw), as can be seen in Charles Quint (Charles V, ruler of the Holy Roman Empire), Archduke Rudolf II of Austria, Ferdinand II of Hungary and Bohemia, and Philip IV of Spain (Fig. 59). Philip IV and his daughter, Margaret Theresa, are the subjects of Velazquez's *Las Meninas* (Fig. 40), although the king himself is seen only in the reflection in a mirror behind the painter. In Velazquez's painting, the young princess does not appear to have the typical jawline, but later portraits of her clearly show her heritage. This form of prognathism, which is autosomal dominant (with variable penetrance) is now referred to as "Habsburg jaw."[27] Philip IV's son, Charles II of Spain, had the most pronounced

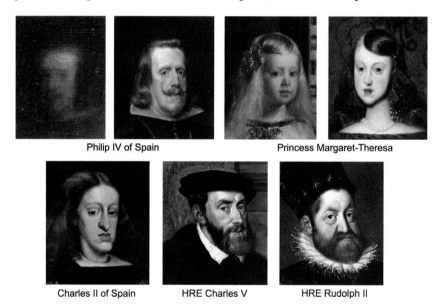

Philip IV of Spain   Princess Margaret-Theresa

Charles II of Spain   HRE Charles V   HRE Rudolph II

Fig. 59: A few members of the Habsburg dynasty, exhibiting the typical eponymous prognathism. A: Diego Velazquez, Mirror reflection in the painting in Fig. 40, of a portrait he painted the same year; B: Young Princess Margaret-Theresa, daughter of Philip IV, detail from Fig. 40. She did not exhibit the typical family jaw until later, as seen in C: Presumed student of Velazquez, 1662–64. *Bottom left:* Juan Carreño de Miranda, circa 1685; *middle:* Titian, circa 1550; *right:* Joseph Heintz the Elder, circa 1592. (HRE: Holy Roman Emperor)

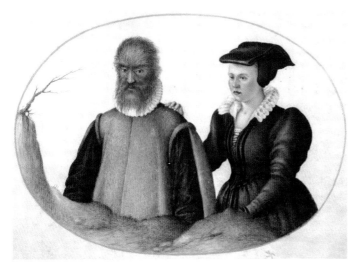
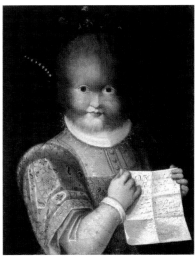

form of the condition, leading to extreme prognathism, near-inability to close his mouth, drooling, and associated mental disorder, likely a result of inbreeding (Fig. 59).[28] His sterility contributed to the extinction of that branch of the family.[29] In the absence of descendants of the Spanish Habsburgs or their genetic material, knowledge about the condition and its pattern of inheritance is derived solely from the hundreds of regal portraits.[30]

A syndrome or disorder can be associated with art in other ways as well. Pedro González (also known as Petrus Gonsalvus) was born in Tenerife in the sixteenth century. He was afflicted with hypertrichosis, or hirsutism (Fig. 60). His life story is well chronicled, as is his family's: four of his seven children were similarly afflicted (Fig. 61), suggesting the diagnosis of this autosomal dominant condition.[31] The condition is also called Ambras syndrome, after the Chamber of Art and Curiosities in Ambras castle in Innsbruck, Austria, where portraits of the González family and other patients afflicted with hypertrichosis are exhibited. The condition is also referred to, pejoratively, as werewolf syndrome. It has been suggested that the fairy tale of "Beauty and the Beast" was based on Pedro and his wife Catherine, but most historians believe that variants of the tale are at least thousands of years old. However, Jean Marais's version of the Beast in the 1946 Jean Cocteau film was inspired by González's portrait.[32]

A particularly vivid example of art intersecting with medicine is Angelman disease, and its obsolete description of "happy puppet syndrome." The syndrome is caused by a deletion or other mutation in the PW/AS region on the long arm of chromosome 15. Patients with this condition are developmentally delayed; they tend to have a happy

Fig. 60: Joris Hoefnagel, *Pedro González and His Wife, Catherine,* circa 1575.

Fig. 61: Lavinia Fontana, *Antonietta Gonsalvus,* 1595, afflicted by hirsutism like her father and three other siblings.

personality and balance problems, often displaying jerky movements. The syndrome is named after Harry Angelman, a British pediatrician who first described several children with the disorder.[33] He called the condition "Happy puppet syndrome" after seeing Caroto's painting of *Boy with a Puppet* in Verona (Fig. 62, bottom right).[34] The term *happy puppet syndrome* is no longer used as it is considered to be derogatory.

There is an additional link between art and medicine for this particular chromosomal anomaly: Angelman syndrome is caused by a gene defect in the maternal copy of a gene on chromosome 15; unlike

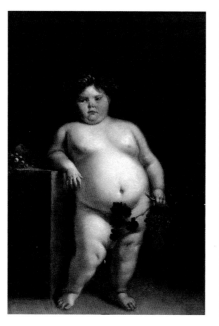
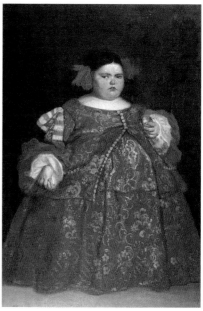
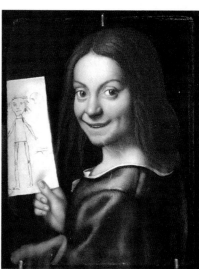

Fig. 62: Example of genomic imprinting: same genetic defect (abnormal allele on chromosome 15), but different phenotype, depending on whose abnormal allele it is—mother or father. *Above left and right:* possible Prader-Willi syndrome, as suggested by Andrea Prader himself. Juan Carreño de Miranda, Portraits of Eugenia Martinez Vallejo, sometimes titled *La Monstrua desnuda* (The nude monster) and *vestida* (clothed), circa 1680; *right:* Giovanni Caroto, *Ritratto di Giovane con Disegno Infantile* (Portrait of a boy with a childish drawing), sixteenth century. The painting of a happy child with a drawing of a puppet inspired Angelman to call his disease "happy puppet syndrome," a now obsolete moniker.

most autosomal disorders, where it does not matter whose gene copy (mother or father) is the defective one, this condition is an example of genomic imprinting: if the paternal allele of that same gene region on chromosome 15 is defective, the phenotype of the disease is completely different.[35] The most characteristic aspect of this disorder, which was described by the Swiss physicians Andrea Prader and Heinrich Willi, is a disruption in the satiety center of the brain, leading to overeating and morbid obesity (in addition to a short stature and developmental delay). It is said that Andrea Prader, while visiting the Prado Museum in Madrid, recognized "his syndrome" in *La Monstrua* (another pejorative name), two portraits by Juan Carreño de Miranda, one clothed and one nude, of a young girl named Eugenia Martinez Vallejo (Fig. 62).[36]

In some cases, an artist is directly associated with a disorder. Such is the case with Toulouse-Lautrec syndrome. Henri de Toulouse-Lautrec was an influential artist of the late nineteenth century in Paris (Fig. 63) and, like Auguste Renoir, Édouard Manet, Edgar Degas, and others before them, a prolific chronicler of Parisian life. But where Degas painted horse races at Longchamp and ballet dancers at the Opéra de Paris, Toulouse-Lautrec preferred the more lowbrow entertainment of the Folies-Bergères, the Moulin Rouge, and other cabarets where cancan dancers and vaudeville artists performed for rowdy crowds. He left us many paintings and drawings (see Fig. 85), and is equally famous for his lithographs and posters, which were used to advertise such celebrities of the era as Aristide Bruant, Jane Avril, and Louise Weber, better known under her stage name of La Goulue. As famously portrayed in popular culture (photographs, biopics), Toulouse-Lautrec was of very short stature, caused by severely foreshortened legs (his head and torso were of normal proportions). He was known to have fractured both femurs as a child, and the fractures never healed properly. More than fifty years after his death, it was first argued that he suffered from picno-dysostosis, a hereditary condition that is autosomal recessive—that is, it is manifested only if both parents are carriers of the abnormal gene.[37] Toulouse-Lautrec's parents were first cousins, and consanguinity greatly enhances the risk of having offspring with a recessive disorder. The condition affects long bones predominantly and is related to osteogenesis imperfecta and achondroplasia (the most common and most recognizable form of congenital dwarfism).

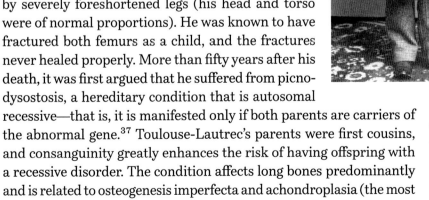

Fig. 63: Henri de Toulouse-Lautrec, 1882.

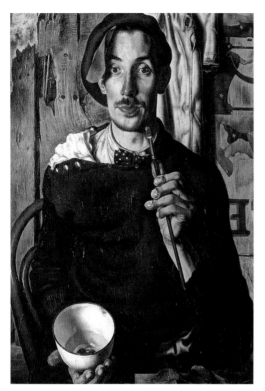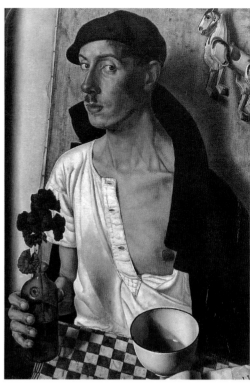

Fig. 64: Dick Ket, self-portraits, *left:* 1939; *right:* 1932. Note the clubbed fingers and acrocyanosis: blueish discoloration of lips and nailbeds, signs of congenital heart disease.

Not many artists can claim to have a disease named after them, but some (like Gerard de Lairesse) have become poster children for the condition that may have afflicted them. As medical knowledge has advanced, more recent artists and their works have offered increasingly clear descriptions of their condition. Dick Ket was a Dutch painter of the early twentieth century. His style is often characterized as magic realism, although his earlier work was influenced mostly by the Impressionists. He left us numerous self-portraits that demonstrate very characteristic features (Fig. 64): dark, bluish-red lips, blue fingernails, and, most dramatically, clubbed fingers. This condition is also called *hippocratisme digital* in French (as it is believed to have been recognized by Hippocrates himself) and is a result of chronic lack of oxygen to the peripheral tissues. Although clubbed fingers can be seen in other conditions, such as severe, chronic lung disease, it is most typical of a specific class of congenital heart anomalies called cyanotic heart diseases, the most common of which is Tetralogy of Fallot. Regardless of the exact etiology, the end result is that nonoxygenated blood, which is supposed to be directed toward the lungs to be oxygenated, bypasses the right side of the heart and ends up instead on the left side, and from there in the aorta and the systemic circulation. As a result, all tissues of the body receive poorly oxygenated blood, giving a bluish hue to the body parts that are the farthest from the heart, such as the fingertips, a sign called acrocyanosis, or blue extremities. The clubbing of the fingertips is likely a result of increased blood vessel density to compensate for the lack of oxygen carried by the blood, which in turn stimulates soft tissue growth. However, the exact mechanism is not known.

Dick Ket suffered from a weak constitution throughout his entire life, living reclusively in his parents' home. The features of cyanosis are recognizable in all his self-portraits. It was therefore not a late finding, as would be seen with progressive lung diseases such as bronchiectasis or chronic obstructive pulmonary disease (COPD), but rather a condition he had his entire life. Although there is no radiologic or autopsy evidence of the exact diagnosis, it is generally accepted that Ket was born with Tetralogy of Fallot[38] (also referred to as blue baby syndrome) or another form of cyanotic heart disease, such as (compensated) transposition of the great vessels.[39] He died in 1940, days shy of his thirty-eighth birthday and three years before Alfred Blalock, Vivien Thomas, and Helen Taussig developed the procedure at Johns Hopkins Hospital that would save the lives of countless "blue babies," a shunt between the subclavian artery and the pulmonary artery beyond the level of the obstruction, allowing more blood to flow to the lungs to be oxygenated. The landmark 1945 paper in the *Journal of the American Medical Association* (*JAMA*)[40] is richly illustrated by artists in the Department of Arts as Applied to Medicine at Johns Hopkins University, the school that Max Brödel built (Fig. 65). Dick Ket is of course not the only person to have been affected by cyanotic heart disease, or even the only (semi-) famous one. But his extraordinary talent and honesty have produced vivid images of the disease that rival any textbook photograph.

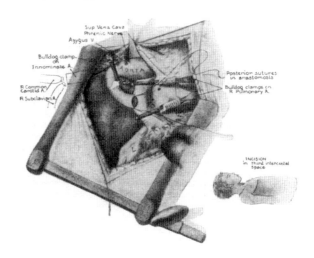

Fig. 65: Illustration of the Blalock-Taussig shunt to treat blue baby syndrome, published in 1945. (Reproduced with permission from *JAMA* 1984, Volume 252, No. 16, p. 2124. Copyright © 1984 American Medical Association. All rights reserved.)

Visionary or Impaired Vision?

When artists are ill, it can affect their art. That may be interesting information for the viewer, but it can also serve to understand the disease itself. A gifted artist, like an eloquent patient, can make it easier for a doctor to help him or her. Objective physical examination is crucial, of course, but so is good history-taking. An unreliable narrator, by contrast, can make the task of the physician more difficult. Of course, the subjective view of the patient can provide insight into a psychiatric malady. Whether it is the interpretation of hallucinations or the visual expression of chronic pain, the patient's voice is not only important to the compassionate physician, but it can teach doctors firsthand about how diseases are experienced.

Like Dick Ket's, the medical history of Frida Kahlo has been well chronicled.[41] At the age of twenty-four, she suffered a horrific injury

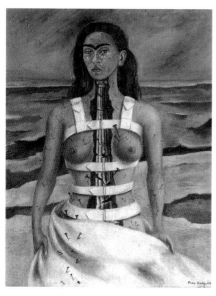

Fig. 66: Frida Kahlo, *La Columna Rota* (The broken column), 1944.

while riding a city bus: a penetrating wound of the abdomen that pierced through her pelvis, in addition to several broken vertebrae and several other fractures. She spent months in the hospital, underwent many painful operations, and continued to suffer from chronic back pain for many years. Her experiences are vividly rendered in several paintings in which she observes how her own body fails her, mutilated by steel rods, screws, and other hardware (Fig. 66). In one painting, she depicts herself as an "Aztec" and a "European" Frida with a detailed portrayal of a blood transfusion, a practice that had not become widespread until only a decade or two earlier. These are obviously not medical illustrations, but they do illustrate how the world of a chronic sufferer can be colored by their disease: they teach us to better understand our patients, the better to take care of them.

For a visual artist, vision is everything, of course. Any condition that affects the eye, or the perception of images, will influence the graphic artist's work. In rare cases, the artist's view of the world gives us an opportunity to witness the effects of a particular medical condition firsthand. As they faithfully reproduce what they see, their paintings demonstrate the pathophysiology of their disease more vividly than a medical dissertation. Thus, what may have been meant to be art for art's sake becomes an educational tool, a way for medical students or doctors in training to better understand the disease, and to better understand their patients' experience.

Of course, visual art is all about how artists interpret what they see, the technique they want to utilize, the message they want to convey, and how innovative they want to be. Is a nonfigurative painting a result of the artist's distorted vision, altered perception of a faithful image,

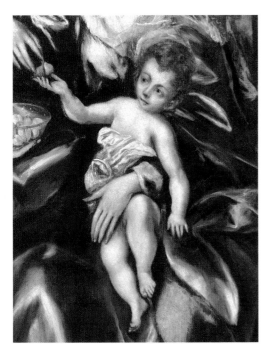

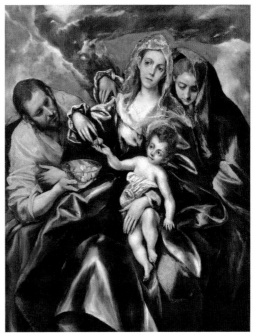

or stylistic liberties? Take El Greco (Doménikos Theotokópoulos), for example. When considered out of context, the figure of Jesus in his *Holy Family with Mary Magdalen* (Fig. 67) may have features of Cornelia de Lange syndrome, a congenital disorder that affects many organ systems.[42] Children with Cornelia de Lange syndrome have a characteristic appearance: arched, thick eyebrows, large irregular ears, a long flat philtrum, a smooth upper lip, and a small jaw. They often have limb anomalies, such as missing or fused fingers (syndactyly). (The widow's peak, seen in Fig. 67, is not typical of Cornelia de Lange syndrome.) However, when we look at his entire oeuvre, we realize that that is how El Greco tended to paint people—long, thin faces with sharp noses and protruding ears (Fig. 68). Of course, one could argue that El Greco had an eyesight problem, precisely because all his characters have elongated features: someone even suggested that this was due to the painter's astigmatism, a condition caused by an abnormally curved cornea or lens, which causes a distorted view of objects. This diagnosis has been attributed to Amedeo Modigliani as well.[43] However, Nobel laureate Dr. Peter Medawar has pointed out, in his "El Greco test" argument, that someone afflicted with astigmatism, or any other eye condition that distorts shapes, would reproduce them correctly: if El Greco saw a circle as an elongated oval, he would have painted what looked like an oval to him and therefore a circle to us.[44]

Left: Fig. 67: Doménikos Theotokópoulos, known as El Greco, *The Holy Family with Mary Magdalen* (detail), circa 1595. The figure of Jesus has thick, arched eyebrows, large irregular ears, a small jaw, and his fingers are weirdly crossed. To some, it is reminiscent of the features of Cornelia de Lange syndrome.

Right: Fig. 68: Same as Fig. 67, full painting. It is clear that long, thin figures with sharp features were El Greco's style.

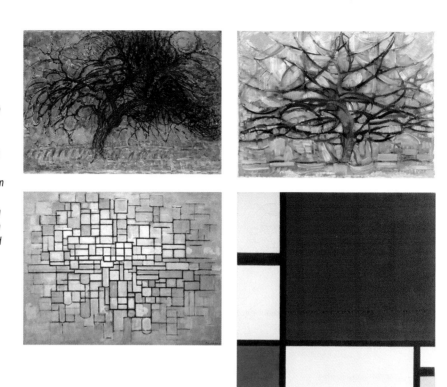

Fig. 69: Piet Mondrian, *top left to right: Avond; De Rode Boom* (Evening; The red tree), 1908–10; *top right: De Grijze Boom* (The gray tree), 1911; *bottom left: Composition No. 11 (Composition in Blue, Gray, and Pink),* 1913; *bottom right: Composition with Red, Blue, and Yellow,* 1930.

At times, the gradual change in style is a sign of the artist's journey. Piet Mondrian, who is famous for his black, rectangular frames colored with red, yellow, white, and blue patches, started out with figurative paintings of rural scenes and in particular the intricate crisscrossing of the branches of trees in winter. The evolution from recognizable trees to abstract lines is clearly a stylistic choice, not a result of Mondrian's altered eyesight (Fig. 69).[45]

But what if the style evolution of an artist was in fact due to worsening vision? Researchers have argued exactly that to explain Edgar Degas's later paintings. We know that the painter developed a retinopathy (mostly in his right eye). A team of ophthalmologists, led by Michael Marmor, estimated the effect that the progressive macular disease may have had on Degas's eyesight.[46] One of his go-to topics was a woman's morning toilet, and he has left us countless variations on the theme, spread out over decades. Early on, the features are fine and detailed, and the broad strokes rendering the skin are smooth (Fig. 70). A decade or so later, the theme has not changed, but the style is wilder, less precise, and the flesh tones are streaked and coarse (Fig. 71). Marmor et al. argue that, to Degas's diminishing eyesight, these strokes would not have appeared coarse at all (agreeing with Medawar's El Greco test). His decreased vision would have caused a

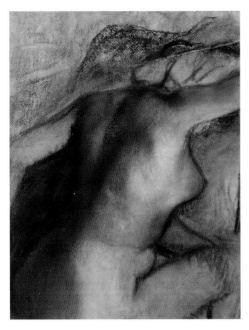
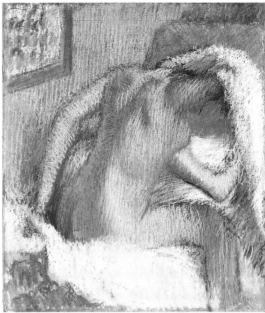

blur, making these streaks appear smooth, at least to him. That this was not a deliberate evolution can be confirmed, according to them, by the fact that Degas never mentioned any desire to experiment or alter his style, whereas he often commented on his gradual loss of vision. Furthermore, they say, the later drawings and paintings were created on much larger sheets of paper, suggesting that he could no longer master fine, meticulous technique. They quote art critic Paul-André Lemoisne, who, in his five-volume catalog of the painter's work, *Degas et son Oeuvre* (Degas and his works), observed that these were "tragic witnesses of the battle of the artist against his infirmity."

Claude Monet, too, suffered from an ophthalmic condition—bilateral cataracts. His annoyance at, and later suffering from, the progressive diminution of his eyesight is well documented in his letters and in reports from friends who urged him to be treated. Clouding of the lens causes a progressive blurring of the visual field, and a gradual change in color perception: reds and oranges predominate, and it becomes more difficult to discern blue and purple tones. In the same 2006 article that discusses Degas's ophthalmic woes, Marmor argues that the progressive clouding of Monet's lenses can be seen in his paintings, particularly the repetitious compositions of lily pads and willow trees on a pond.[47] The 1899 painting of a bridge over a pond has a generally blue-green color scheme. The lilies, pond grass, and trees in the background are remarkably detailed, despite the Impressionist style (Fig. 72). In contrast, a very similar composition

Fig. 70: Edgar Degas, *La Toilette*, 1885.

Fig. 71: Edgar Degas, *Woman Drying Her Hair*, 1900–1908.

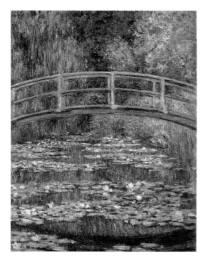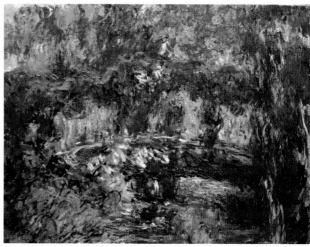

Fig. 72: Claude
Monet, *Bridge over
a Pond of Water
Lilies*, 1899.

Fig. 73: Claude
Monet, *The
Japanese Bridge*,
1920–22. Brown
and orange colors
predominate, and
the scenery lacks
detail, possibly a
result of the artist's
poor eyesight from
bilateral cataracts.

around 1922 shows an overwhelmingly orange-brown composition and blurry shadows representing the footbridge and the trees (Fig. 73). Of course, this may have been a deliberate stylistic choice, and the color of the leaves may just reflect an autumnal scenery. But, argues Marmor, Monet's last paintings would contradict that.

In 1923, at the age of eighty-three and after incessant pressure from his friends, he finally agreed to undergo cataract surgery. (Cataract surgery, whereby the clouded lens is removed altogether, was even then a relatively benign and safe procedure, as illustrated in Fig. 38.) A painting of a pond with lilies and willow trees, which he completed in 1826, shows a style that is very reminiscent of his 1899 painting, with exquisite details and a palette that is again predominantly green and blue (Fig. 74).[48]

As in the conspiracy theories around Vincent van Gogh (see later), the argument that Monet's alleged cataracts had an effect on his art relies in part on cherry-picking examples from his oeuvre: when looking at all his water lily–inspired paintings, it is clear that he had experimented for decades. In his well-known series of paintings of haystacks in the field or Chartres cathedral, he was recreating the effect of light at various times during the day and throughout the seasons. Similarly, some reddish-orange versions of the water lily ponds and tree-lined lanes long predate his deteriorating eyesight, while other, greener landscapes date from well into the 1920s, when his cataracts were supposedly at their worst. Claude Monet is long gone, and he cannot tell us what happened to him. A more recent story bears remarkable resemblance to Monet's experience, however. Yvonne Fuller, a medical illustrator for the *British Medical Journal* before she retired, chronicled her own troubles with cataracts, and how surgery restored her vision. A watercolorist, she

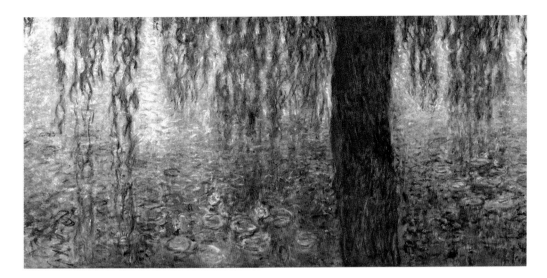

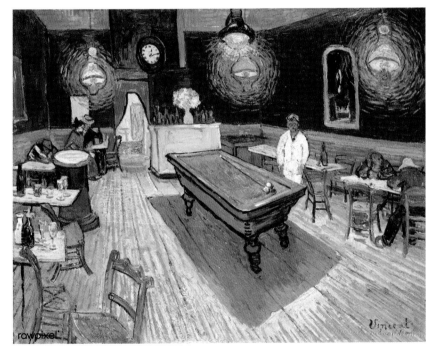

Fig. 74: Claude Monet, *Nymphéas* (Water lilies) (detail), completed in 1926. Painted in the last year of his life, after he had undergone cataract surgery, the colors blue and green predominate, and the lily flowers and willow leaves are more detailed, reminiscent of his earlier work before he developed cataracts.

Fig. 75: Vincent van Gogh, *The Night Café*, 1888. This is one of van Gogh's paintings, with halos around the light sources, that helped spread a rumor that the artist suffered from glaucoma. (Photo by Rawpixel, licensed under CC BY-SA 4.)

painted examples of how images were blurred, objects were duplicated, and browns and oranges dominated until she had one eye and then the other treated. After her cataract operations, her vision returned to normal, as beautifully demonstrated by before-and-after paintings she made of the same coastal landscape:[49] reminiscent of what she used to see before her operations, she shows how the multiple blurry sails and yellow-orange landscape seen through clouded lenses are really only a single boat under a bright blue sky.

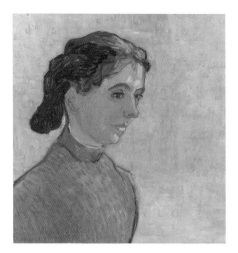
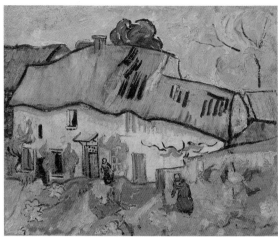

Fig. 76: Vincent van Gogh, *left: The Little Arlésienne; right: Landscape with Three Trees and a House,* 1890.

Despite convincing arguments, Degas's and Monet's alleged vision problems remain suppositions, just like the theories (bordering on conspiracies) around the work of Vincent van Gogh. As with Frida Kahlo, whose physical and psychological trauma is present in her paintings, van Gogh's mental illness is said to have influenced his art, particularly in his later years.[50] Some have also speculated on the origin of concentric circles around bright lights in some of his paintings, such as *Starry Night* and *The Night Café* (Fig. 75). Was his vision affected by glaucoma?[51] Glaucoma is a condition characterized by increased pressure inside the globe, which in severe and chronic forms can lead to blindness. In moderately severe forms, it changes the way the eye captures an image, and it can alter the perception of color and blur an image. It also worsens the perception of light intensity and creates halos around bright lights. Then again, it is entirely possible that the halos around the stars in van Gogh's painting are an expression of artistic license—Impressionism was all about exploring the way the world is perceived by the artist rather than the realism of naturalistic art. Thomas Lee and his colleagues noted something else about van Gogh, however, particularly during the period in 1890 when he left Arles, in the south of France, to move to Auvers to be closer to his brother Theo and Dr. Gachet, who cared for him.[52] Many of the paintings in that period have a distinct yellow hue (Fig. 76). Lee floated the idea, in a 1981 scientific article, that this may have been a result of digoxin intoxication. Digoxin is a potent drug extracted from the purple or woolly foxglove (*Digitalis purpurea* and *Digitalis lanata,* respectively), bright purple or white flowers that grow freely in most temperate regions around the world. The medicinal uses of the foxglove had been known for centuries. Digitalis is a cardiac gly-

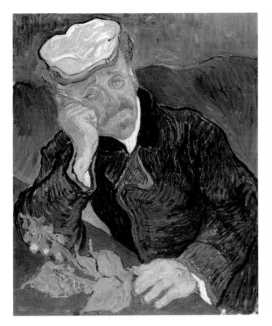 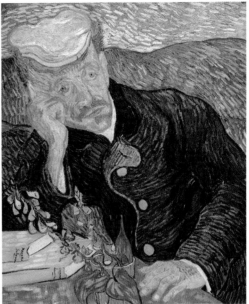

coside that was the first effective treatment for heart failure as early as 1930. However, its use in medicine predates the discovery of its cardiac effects. At one time, it was used to treat epilepsy and other mental conditions. We don't know whether Dr. Gachet used digitalis to treat van Gogh's afflictions, but we know that he grew foxglove and many other medicinal plants and herbs in the garden adjacent to his house, where van Gogh was a guest and patient.

Digitalis is a drug with a very narrow therapeutic margin: the effective dose is very close to toxic levels. Patients with a digitalis intoxication often suffer from xanthopsia—seeing yellow. (This is very different from jaundice, which makes the patient look, not see, yellow. In severe jaundice, or icterus, even the white of the eye (the sclera) looks yellow, but that doesn't mean the patient experiences a change in color perception.) In xanthopsia, everything appears yellow to the patient. The suggestion that van Gogh's paintings during that period may have been influenced by a visual impairment secondary to digitalis intoxication is strengthened, according to Lee, by the fact that the only two portraits he painted of Dr. Gachet show him clutching a bunch of foxgloves (Fig. 77).[53] Then again, at least one of these portraits is notable for its deep blue colors, undermining the xanthopsia theory. Moreover, many of van Gogh's famous paintings, such as *The Night Café* (Fig. 75), *Sunflowers,* and *The Yellow House* (in Arles) (Fig. 78), are predominantly yellow, yet all predate his treatment by Dr. Gachet.[54] "Si non e vero, e bene trovato," the conspiracy theory behind van Gogh's yellow palette,

Fig. 77: Vincent van Gogh, Two portraits of Dr. Gachet, 1890. In both, the doctor clutches a bunch of foxglove flowers. Digitalis, a cardiac drug, is extracted from the purple foxglove (*Digitalis purpurea*). Digitalis overdose can cause xanthopsia (seeing yellow).

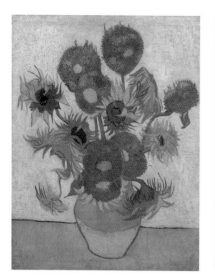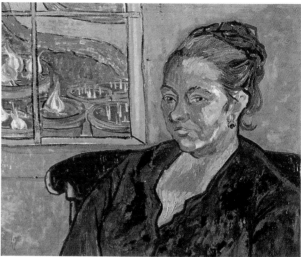

Fig. 78: Vincent van Gogh's yellow palette, all predating his alleged period of xanthopsia in 1890. *Left: Sunflowers,* 1889; *right: Portrait of Augustine Roulin,* 1888.

may be just that, but it is still a vivid way to demonstrate xanthopsia to medical students.

In a peculiar coincidence that unites art, medicine, and medical illustration, digitalis is also at the origin of Dr. Frank Netter's career. The most recognizable name in modern anatomic and medical illustration was approached by the CIBA pharmaceutical company in 1936 as they were launching their version of digoxin.[55] The full-color pamphlet showed a superbly detailed illustration of the outside of a heart; the inside of the brochure showed an equally beautiful rendering of the interior of the cardiac chambers. The ad campaign was so successful that CIBA commissioned more illustrations from Netter, and this decades-long collaboration led to his magnum opus, the eight-volume *CIBA Collection of Medical Illustrations.*

The theories of how visual impairment influenced the art of van Gogh, Degas, and even Monet are intriguing but impossible to prove. In the case of Edvard Munch, however, we know because he described it himself repeatedly. Munch was one of the most prominent representatives of the Expressionist movement and is best known for his iconic *The Scream,* the haunting portrait of a grotesque person with a distorted face, seemingly screaming amid a nightmarish, postapocalyptic landscape. He was much more than that, however, and was a prolific avant-garde artist who left us thousands of drawings, etchings, watercolors, and oil paintings, including *The Inheritance* (Fig. 50). In 1930, he developed a scotoma, a large blind spot within the visual field that can be the result of vitreous hemorrhage or retinal detachment. If left untreated, retinal detachment becomes progressively worse and leads to blindness, and in Munch's time, treatment did not exist. (Today, retinal

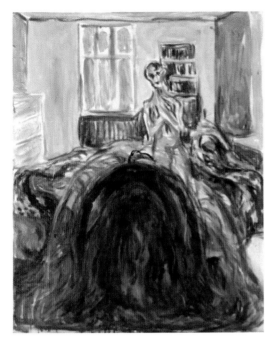
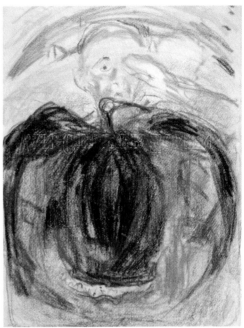

detachment can be stopped, or even reversed, using laser surgery.) The fact that Munch regained full vision a year or so later suggests that his scotoma was not a sign of retinal detachment, but there is no doubt that he experienced symptoms.[56] Not only did he describe the feeling in letters to his friends, but he used his visual impairment as a way to experiment. In a series of pen-and-ink sketches, crayon drawings, and oil paintings, he features his blind spot "front and center." In one piece, the room can be seen only peripherally as the central portion of the painting is black (Fig. 79); in two other works, he transforms the black spot into a bird, adding a beak and feathers (Fig. 80). Munch later developed similar scotomas in his other eye, and eventually learned to harness his visual impairment to further his art.

Fig. 79: Edvard Munch, *Disturbed Vision,* 1930. Self-portrait with a prominent, central scotoma (dark spot), an ophthalmic condition he incorporated in the painting.

Fig. 80: Edvard Munch, *The Artist's Injured Eye (and a Figure of a Bird's Head),* 1930. Munch experiments with using the blind spot in the center of his field of vision as part of the painting, turning the scotoma into a bird.

Medical Selfies

If Munch chronicled his ailments in his paintings, at least two other artists used their talents as gifted illustrators to advance the treatment of their condition. Sometime between 1509 and 1521, the famous German painter and engraver Albrecht Dürer suffered from abdominal pain, and sent his physician a self-portrait in which he indicated his condition (Fig. 81). In what can be considered the first medical selfie, Dürer drew a self-portrait, showing him pointing at a spot in his upper-

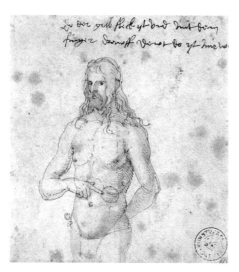

Fig. 81: Albrecht Dürer, *Selbstbildnis, Krank* (Self-portrait, sick), also known as *The Sick Dürer*, circa 1510, a self-portrait the artist allegedly sent to an out-of-town physician to explain where his pain was. The inscription says "There, where the yellow spot is and where I point my finger, is where it hurts."

left quadrant, with the caption "There, where the yellow mark is and where I'm pointing, is where it hurts." It is not known which condition Dürer was suffering from, or whether the doctor, who lived hundreds of miles away, was able to cure him. Not many conditions give rise to left upper abdominal pain. Geoffrey Schott has argued that Dürer could have suffered from malaria, and that pain in the left upper quadrant could be a result of splenic infarction or abscess.[57] However, right upper quadrant pain and tenderness are quite common and most often caused by gallstones or liver conditions. It is probably too much of a stretch to suggest that Dürer, while drawing his self-portrait, forgot that he was looking in the mirror and may have confused his left with his right.

Centuries later, Max Brödel, the medical illustrator at Johns Hopkins Hospital, suffered an injury to his left arm while doing research and cutting himself on a fragment of pelvic bone from a patient who had died of generalized streptococcal sepsis. The wound became infected and caused nerve damage. He required intense treatment and was tended by his friend and collaborator, Harvey Cushing, the famed Johns Hopkins neurosurgeon. While hospitalized at the Johns Hopkins Hospital, Brödel described the pattern of his symptoms in the best way he knew: by drawing his left arm and hand in the hospital chart, indicating which parts of his limb were numb. This detailed description corresponds perfectly to the innervation of the ulnar nerve, confirming Cushing's diagnosis. He ultimately recovered, documenting the progressive return of sensation in his arm in successive drawings.[58]

Max Brödel is considered the father of modern medical illustration, codifying its core principles and starting its very first educational program. Although his ideas are still very relevant today, he lived and practiced more than a century ago, and a lot has changed in medicine. Through his illustrations, as well those of contemporary artists who were not necessarily medical illustrators, we learn a lot about the history of modern medicine and surgery. Paintings representing famous doctors of the day may not qualify as medical illustration any more than the occasional depiction of disease in classical art, but insofar as history can teach us a lot about who we are, glimpses of nineteenth-century medical practices can teach us where we came from.

Art shows us the mores of the era in which it was produced, including the medical practices of its time. It shows us the evolution of the medical profession in ways that are complementary to medical illustration, and the two disciplines sometimes overlap.[59] The renowned American painter Thomas Eakins produced large paintings, fourteen years apart, of two of the greatest surgeons in Philadelphia. *The Gross Clinic,* completed in 1875, shows Professor Samuel D. Gross as he demonstrates one of his operations (Fig. 82). There are more than thirty people around him—assistants, colleagues, students—all men and all dressed in street clothes. Louis Pasteur had published his findings on

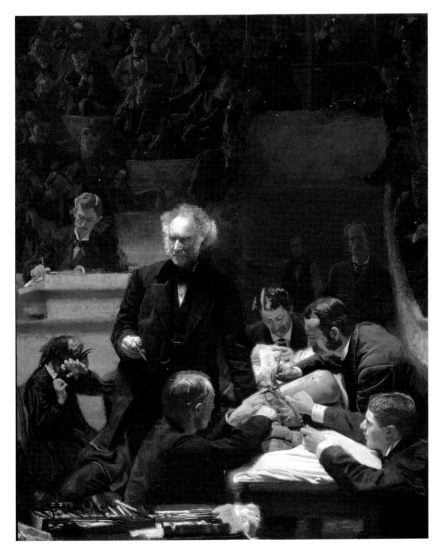

Fig. 82: Thomas Eakins, *Portrait of Dr. Samuel D. Gross (The Gross Clinic),* 1875.

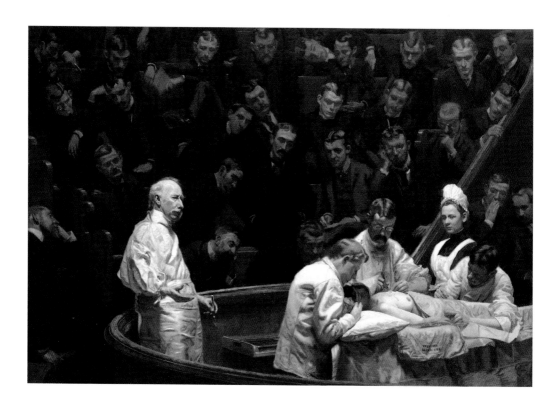

Fig. 83: Thomas
Eakins, *The Agnew
Clinic*, 1889.

microorganisms in 1861, and Joseph Lister had introduced the principles of asepsis in 1867, but these concepts had not yet been widely
applied to hospitals and operating theaters. Fourteen years later, *The
Agnew Clinic* tells a different story: The protagonists all wear white,
and while they are still predominantly men, there is one very important
female figure, positioned opposite Dr. Agnew, and equally authoritative
in her stance—the head nurse, ushering the era of modern collabora-
tive healthcare where doctors, surgeons, midwives, and nurses work
together (Fig. 83).

Similar changes were seen in Europe. Surgeons like Theodor
Billroth in Germany and Jules-Emile Péan in France performed ever-
more daring abdominal operations (Figs. 84 and 85). (Both surgeons
can rightfully claim to have pioneered the gastrectomy—Péan having
been the first to successfully resect a patient's stomach, and Billroth
having had a patient survive the operation.[60]) Many of these masters
of surgery also helped design increasingly specialized surgical instruments, many of which are still used today and named after them: the
Péan hemostat, the Kocher clamp, the Metzenbaum scissors. These
and other staples of modern surgery are immortalized in many grandiose paintings in the same manner that the masters of anatomy were
portrayed by Rembrandt and others two centuries earlier.

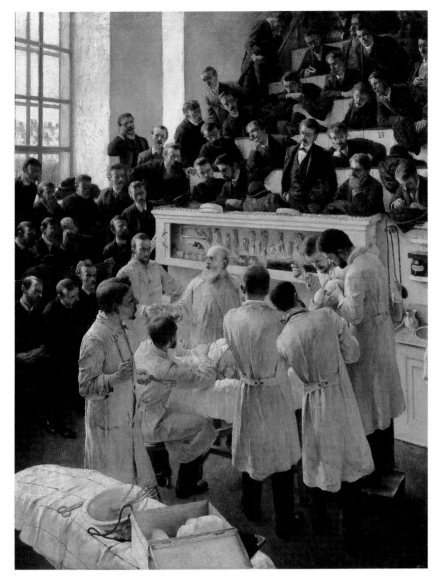

Fig. 84: Adalbert Franz Seligmann, *Theodor Billroth im Hörsaal* (Theodor Billroth operating), 1888–90. Billroth is considered one of the founders of modern abdominal surgery. His many disciples include William Halsted, who mirrored the modern residency training after Billroth's, and Jan Mikulicz-Radecki, who helped popularize the use of surgical gloves, first introduced by Halsted (see Fig. 89).

Success has many fathers: most of the surgical instruments in use today are known by different names, depending on where one practices. The forceps developed by Péan is known in North America as a kelly, after Howard Kelly, the chief of obstetrics and gynecology at Johns Hopkins Hospital who also wrote landmark textbooks on surgery illustrated by Max Brödel. In a clear example of how art, medicine, and medical illustration blend together, the humble surgical clamp (whether a péan or a kelly) is featured in Henri Gervex's painting of Péan, in a caricature of the great French surgeon by Henri de Toulouse-Lautrec (Fig. 85), in an Expressionist painting by Christian Schad (Fig.

Fig. 85: *Left:* Henri Gervex, *Avant l'opération* (Before the operation), 1887. Group portrait with Dr. Jules-Emile Péan. Note the surgical instrument he is holding in his right hand, now known throughout the French-speaking surgical world as a Péan clamp. *Right:* Henri de Toulouse-Lautrec, *Dr. Péan Operating*, 1892. In his right hand, Péan holds his eponymous clamp. (Image courtesy Clark Art Institute. clarkart .edu)

Fig. 86: Christian Schad, *The Operation* (Appendectomy in Geneva), 1929. (Image courtesy of http:// imageofsurgery. com, Fair use.)

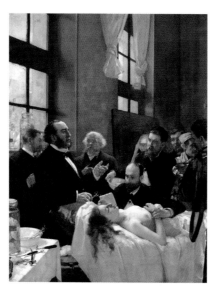

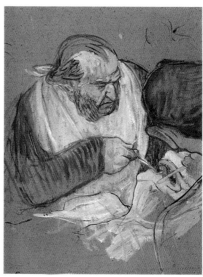

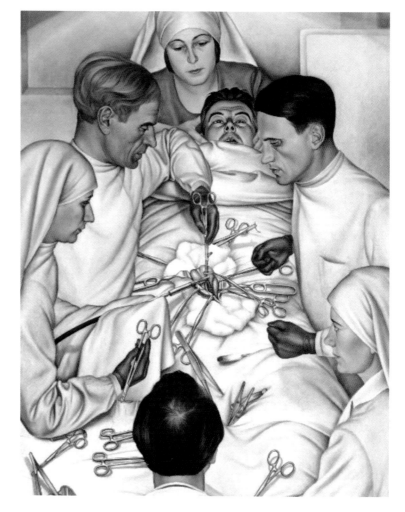

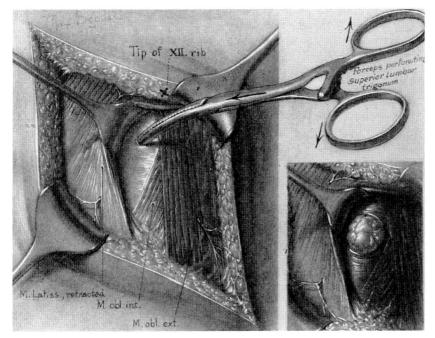

86), as well as in countless medical illustrations, like the one by Max Brödel (Fig. 87).

If classic art is witness to the evolution in medicine, these changes can be found in medical illustration as well. With the wide acceptance of asepsis and the introduction of anesthesia by William Morton in 1846, increasingly complex surgical procedures became possible, and medicine entered the modern era. Surgery occurred in dedicated rooms, rather than in amphitheaters; operative fields were cordoned off with autoclaved cloth drapes; surgeons wore sterile gowns and masks after John Tyndall and Joseph Lister, among others, had shown the existence of airborne germs. To further protect the patient from infection during the operation, the surgeon and his assistants dipped their hands in phenol, or carbolic acid, a very potent antiseptic that is also caustic. In 1890, the chief of surgery at Johns Hopkins Hospital, William Halsted (one of the four physicians who were initially recruited to Baltimore when the hospital was founded), became concerned about the damage that concentrated mercuric chloride (an alternative to phenol) was causing to the hands of his devoted scrub nurse (and later wife), Caroline Hampton.[61] To protect her hands, he ordered latex rubber gloves to be made especially for her. It proved so effective in protecting her hands that soon the other members of the team demanded gloves as well. Thus started the practice of surgical gloves, first at Johns Hopkins Hospital in 1894, and soon throughout the world.[62] In a detailed 1903 medical

Fig. 88: Max Brödel, Renal muscle-splitting incision, in Howard A. Kelly, *Diseases of the Kidneys and Ureters*. Note the ungloved hand as the left fingers guide the incision of the abdominal wall muscles.

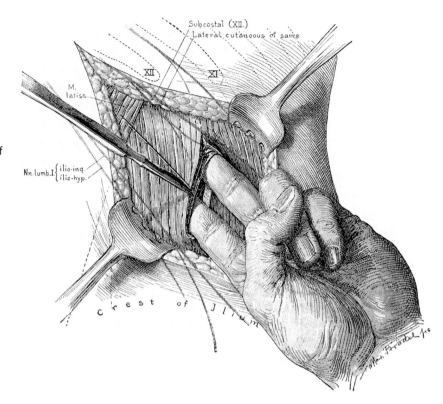

Fig. 89: Max Brödel, Third step in silver wire method of opening kidney, 1922, in Howard A. Kelly, *Diseases of the Kidneys, Ureters and Bladder, with Special Reference to the Diseases of Women*. Surgeons are now wearing latex gloves. Compare this illustration with that in Fig. 88 by the same illustrator, only a few years earlier.

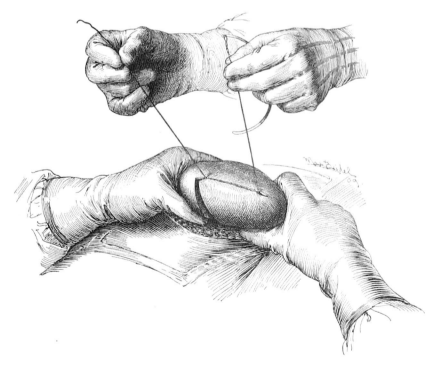

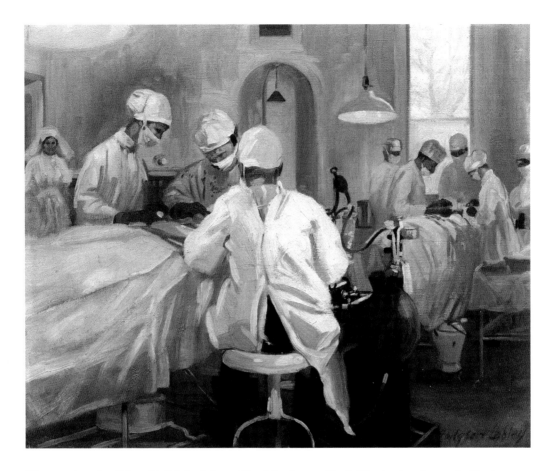

Fig. 90: John Hodgson Lobey, *The Operating Theater*, 1918.

illustration by Max Brödel, Johns Hopkins's medical illustrator-in-residence, one can clearly see the surgeon's bare fingers guide the scalpel as it divides the external oblique muscle to expose the renal fossa (Fig. 88). A similar illustration, a few years later, now shows gloved hands in the operative field (Fig. 89). In addition to the didactic value of detailed medical illustrations, these genuine works of art thus reflect the medical and surgical practices of their time. They offer us a glimpse in the history of the medical specialties. The line between "true art" and medical illustration is often blurred. Both disciplines are witnesses of their time. Jan Mikulicz-Radecki, a famous Polish surgeon, adopted the use of surgical gloves after he visited Halsted in Baltimore. He is also credited with the introduction of surgical masks to further protect patients from their surgeons and vice versa.[63] John Hodgson Lobey's *The Operating Theater* (Fig. 90), which he painted in 1918, shows the entire operating room personnel in surgical gowns, hats, masks, and gloves.[64] In less than fifty years, the way surgery was performed completely changed, and Gross's operating room, as pictured by Eakins (Fig. 82), could not be more different from the scene depicted by Lobey.

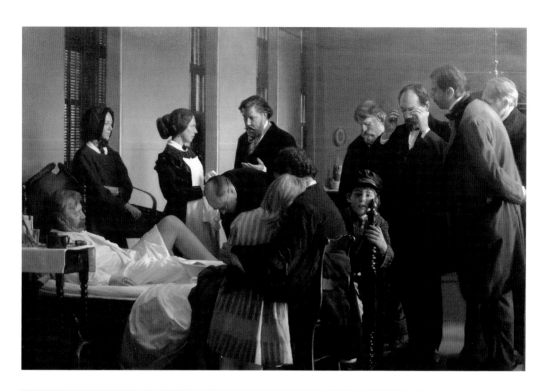

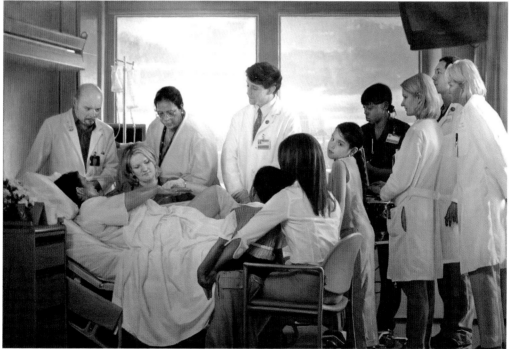

Fig. 91: Warren and Lucia Prosperi, *top:* Rhode Island Hospital 150 years ago; *bottom:* in 2002. (Used by permission of the artists.)

The contemporary artist Warren Prosperi and his wife, renowned photographer Lucia, recreated the seminal event that was the introduction of general anesthesia by Morton. The painting, called *Ether Day,* is displayed prominently at Massachusetts General Hospital, the birthplace of inhalation anesthesia. In a similar vein, and bridging 150 years, Prosperi immortalized the practice of bedside rounds at Rhode Island Hospital in Providence in a manner that emulates Eakins (Fig. 91). The style and composition harken back to last century's medicine, but the dress code and medical paraphernalia in the painting on the right (the hospital bed, the IV poles, and the electronic equipment) are decidedly twenty-first century. The more things change, the more they stay the same.

Chapter 3

The Shady Side of Medical Illustration

There is no clear divide between doctor and patient, or between artist and subject: we are all a part and a product of the world we inhabit. Physicians make decisions that affect other people's lives and must therefore act responsibly, honestly, and without prejudice. Artists and (medical) illustrators may feel like mere observers of the world around them, but they engage with it as well. Their art and their actions can have consequences too.

Controversies in Art

Art can be controversial. In fact, great art is often controversial as artists push boundaries, and the public is not yet ready for whatever the new thing is. In time, we smile at what was once called scandalous or inappropriate: *Le Déjeuner sur l'Herbe* (Luncheon on the grass), Édouard Manet's most famous painting, was rejected by the 1863 Paris Salon (the yearly exhibit of the Académie des Beaux-Arts) more for its "broad brush strokes" than for the scandalous depiction of fully clothed men seemingly oblivious to the naked woman sitting next to them (Fig. 92). Picasso's *Les Demoiselles d'Avignon* (The young ladies of Avignon) was criticized for the grotesque appearance of the women (it heralded the Cubist movement), as well as for the subject—not, as one might think, young ladies from the town of Avignon in the south of France, but prostitutes from a house in the Calle de Aviñón in Barcelona. Both paintings may have touched a similar nerve with

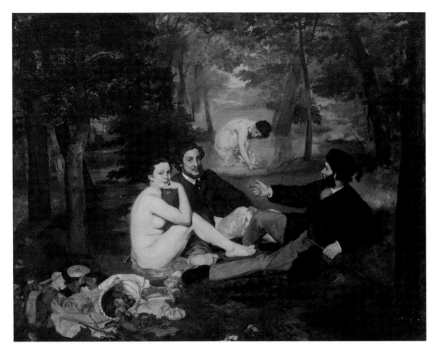

Fig. 92: Édouard Manet, *Le Déjeuner sur l'Herbe* (Luncheon on the grass), 1863.

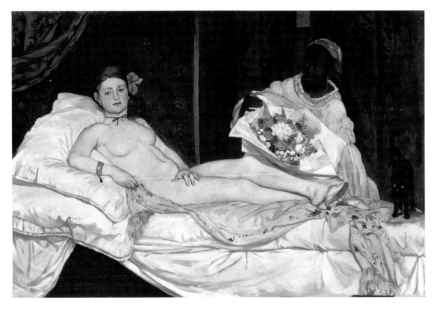

Fig. 93: Édouard Manet, *Olympia*, 1863.

the public, pointing a finger at the hypocrisies of prostitution as an illegal but widely tolerated practice; some have interpreted Manet's piece as set in the Bois de Boulogne, then as now a place known for its offerings of sexual transactions.[1] While nudity is certainly a factor for much scandalous art in history, it was often not the depiction of a naked body itself that caused a stir but the context: the brazen look of Manet's *Olympia* (Fig. 93) or Goya's *La Maja Desnuda* (Naked Maja)

Fig. 94: Francisco
Goya, *La Maja
Desnuda*, (The nude
Maja), circa 1798.

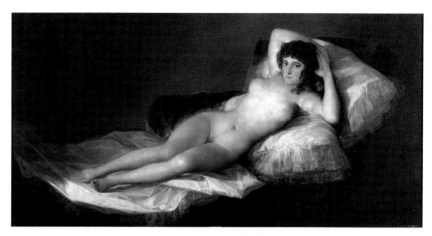

Fig. 95: John Singer
Sargent, *Portrait of
Madame X*, 1884.

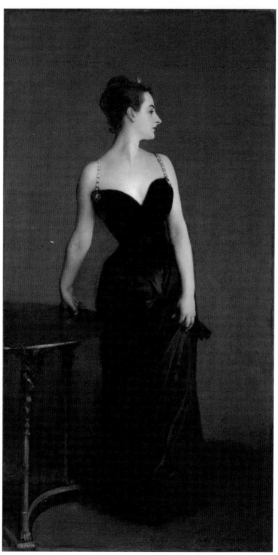

(Fig. 94), who stare unabashedly at the viewer; the dirt on St. Matthew's feet in Caravaggio's 1602 *Saint Matthew and the Angel*;[2] and even John Singer Sargent's Madame X's earlobe, which is too red, evoking lewdness (Fig. 95).[3] It can also be the message, intended or not, that the artist is alluding to. Géricault's *Le Radeau de la* Méduse (The raft of the *Medusa*), showing the shipwrecked passengers of the ship *La Méduse,* abandoned by its crew, purportedly represents the amorality of the government at the time as it neglected the misery of its people.[4] Géricault was not a medical illustrator, of course, but his methods would have made Van Calcar, Richer, Netter, or Brödel proud. For his research into the wretched survivors of the disaster, he painted dismembered bodies at the Paris morgue: anatomic dissections in the tradition of Vesalius and Hunter (Fig. 96).[5]

Medical illustration and the artistic representation of medical subjects have suffered a similar fate. Thomas Eakins's grandiose painting of Dr. Samuel D. Gross (see Fig. 82), which is now prominently displayed at the Philadelphia Museum of Art, was once rejected for display in that very same building (then called Memorial Hall) when it was submitted for the Centennial International Exhibition of 1876. The bloody hand of Dr. Gross, the gruesome operation being performed by his assistants, and the grieving expression of, presumably, the young patient's mother were deemed far too scandalous. It would be simplistic to blame the

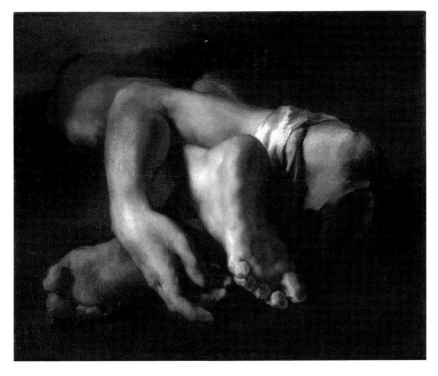

Fig. 96: Théodore Géricault, *Étude de Bras et de Jambes, Peinte à la Lumière de la Lampe* (Study of arms and legs, painted by the light of a lamp), preparatory paintings for *Le Radeau de la* Méduse (The raft of the *Medusa*), 1818–19.

blood and gore for the painting's rejection, however. The museum halls of the world are filled with overly graphic representations of death, disease, war, and destruction, particularly in works of art depicting religious subjects. The anatomy lesson of Dr. Nicolaes Tulp (Fig. 3) is just as graphic as Eakins's painting, and Rembrandt's other anatomy lesson (that of Dr. Deijman, Fig. 97) is much worse. But then Tulp's and Deijman's subjects were executed criminals, while Gross's patient was an innocent child. (In reality, Dr. Gross was demonstrating a conservative operation for osteomyelitis, which, in earlier times, would have required the boy's leg to be amputated.)

Of course, medical illustration as a didactic discipline is not often judged for its gruesome depiction of the body in health and sickness: it is understood that, just like a medical text, it must represent reality in all its ugliness. That doesn't mean that medical illustration has not been plagued by scandals, however. But just like Manet's work was reviled because of its context rather than its models, so too have medical illustrators been questioned about the circumstances surrounding their work rather than the depiction of their subjects. If it seems strange that medical illustrations might bring up ethical questions, consider that, since the beginning of the modern era, medical

Fig. 97: Rembrandt van Rijn, *Anatomische Les van Dr. Jan Deijman* (The anatomy lesson of Dr. Jan Deijman), 1656.

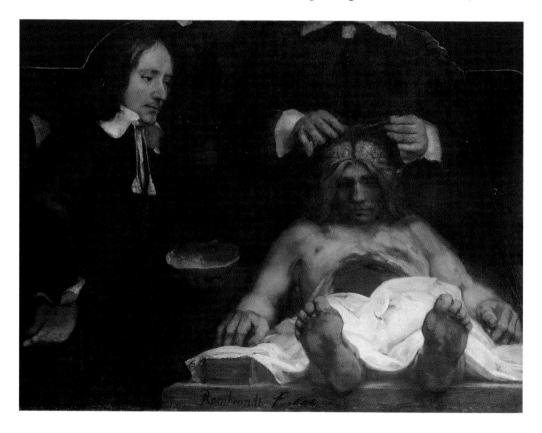

illustration has been intimately associated with anatomic discoveries, and anatomic discoveries have depended heavily on the dissection of human cadavers. While the faithful reproduction of dissected bodies and body parts by illustrators is not brought into question, the provenance of specimens has a somewhat checkered history.

As people sought to understand the internal workings of the body, down and dirty dissections were an obvious must. In ancient societies, where death and disease were much less sanitized and hidden than they are today, the presence of a dead body was not shocking, but the dissection of one was unacceptable. Laws against autopsies in ancient Greece or Egypt may have been dictated by religious tenets,[6] but were likely meant to protect people from diseases carried by putrefaction: not only was medical science in its infancy, but the preservation of dead tissue, other than embalming, would not be possible for another twenty centuries. Thus, Galen, whose teaching prevailed for fourteen hundred years and who is still considered today as one of the greatest physicians of all time, garnered most of his anatomic knowledge from the dissection of animals (dogs and pigs, among others). It is unclear whether he did at times participate in human dissections, but he would not likely have admitted it publicly for fear of retribution.

As mentioned in chapter 2, it is not totally correct to state that the Catholic Church (and authorities in other religions) condemned autopsies. In fact, curiosity about the hidden secrets of the human body reached the church as well, but only in exceptional situations: if some individuals were so inherently good as to deserve beatification or sainthood, surely there must be something that distinguished them from mere mortals?[7] The autopsy of St. Fillipo Neri in the sixteenth century revealed an enormous left ventricle, seen as proof that his heart was full of God's divine love, which helped confirm his sainthood.[8]

In addition to the occasional "pious postmortem," as Brad Bouley calls them,[9] autopsies were also performed to try and explain an unexpected death as far back as the thirteenth century. Of course, only the rich could afford such examination, which was typically done at the home of the deceased. At the other end of the good-bad spectrum, some autopsies may have been performed to confirm a criminal's evil mind. It is important to distinguish between autopsies and human dissections, however. In all cases an autopsy was—and still is—meant to understand the inner workings or pathology of one person.[10] When a human body was dissected for the benefit of acquiring new anatomic knowledge, most ancient societies were less eager to sanction the practice. In the sixteenth century, things began to change as universities flourished, and the pursuit of medical knowledge became more widespread. Vesalius may have been the most important physician-anatomist of his time, but he was far from the only one to perform dissections as part of his lectures. Thus, the need for raw material grew rapidly. Unfortunately, cadavers were not easy to come by as nobody wanted a dearly departed to be desecrated. Human dissection was therefore restricted to criminals and unclaimed bodies, including those of fetuses, newborns, and children in some cases.

Body Snatchers

In 1543, the year his masterpiece was published, Vesalius conducted a public dissection on the body of Jakob Karrer von Gebweiler, a notorious felon in Switzerland. (The so-called "Basel Skeleton" is still on display at the University of Basel.) A century later, a series of group portraits of famed Dutch anatomists echo this practice: in Rembrandt's *De Anatomische Les van Dr. Nicolaes Tulp* (The anatomy lesson of Dr. Nicolaes Tulp), we see the dissection of the forearm muscles of the thief Aris Kindt (Fig. 3).[11] In another painting by Rembrandt, Tulp's successor, Dr. Jan Deijman, is seen dissecting the brain of executed criminal Joris Fonteijn (Fig. 97). And Deijman's successor, Frederik Ruysch, is immortalized in Jan van Neck's painting as he prepares to dissect a stillborn infant, complete with umbilical cord and placenta still attached (Fig. 4). This is probably the first detailed representation of the placenta in art.

As the use of human dissections in medical schools increased, so did the need for "unclaimed" bodies. Noting a slight conflict of interest in the laws of supply and demand, most courts had limited the number of (criminal) bodies that could be dissected by any one university to only a few per year, even as state-sanctioned capital punishment increased across Europe.[12] In England, for example, Henry VIII allowed each university access to four executed felons per year. This was part of the charter recognizing the Company of Barber-Surgeons (Fig. 98) in 1543—that same watershed date in the history of medicine and medical illustration.[13]

While the laws were clear, the legal body-count rules gradually relaxed. However, this was still insufficient to meet the requirements of academic institutions, especially given the popularity of anatomy classes. In eighteenth-century England, William Hunter and his younger brother John owned one of several such schools, primarily catering to the well-to-do but bored London literati. This naturally led to creative ways of procurement. Rather than politely waiting

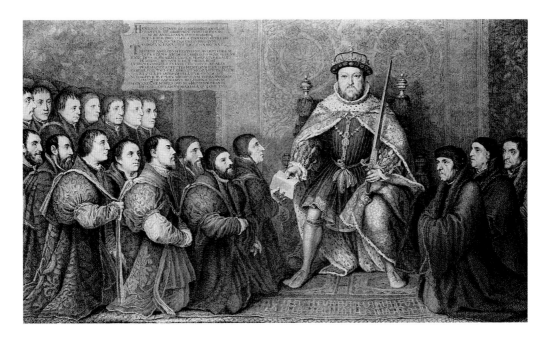

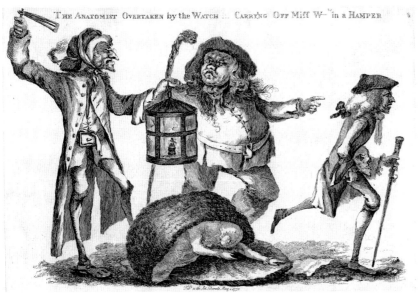

THE ANATOMIST OVERTAKEN by the WATCH ... CARRYING OFF MISS W— in a HAMPER

Above: Fig. 98: Hans Holbein, *Henry VIII and the Barber Surgeons,* 1543.

Left: Fig. 99: William Austin, *The Anatomist Overtaken by the Watch,* 1773. An angry man (center) alerts the Night Watch about a doctor (running away, *right*), who was trying to steal a dead person's body (partially uncovered in the sack abandoned by the body snatcher). (The British Museum, licensed under CC BY-NC-SA 4.0.)

for an unclaimed body, some unsavory individuals, euphemistically called "resurrectionists," resorted to grave robbery.[14] While this was, of course, illegal, it was not often punished harshly. Resurrectionists were in fact less afraid of the arm of the law than the wrath of angry mobs of mourning relatives (Fig. 99). Family members could not stand watch over a grave at all times, and this naturally led to inventive and sometimes lethal methods to protect the departed. These included mortsafes (iron cages placed over a grave), booby-trapped "coffin torpedoes" (US patent #208,672); and so-called cemetery guns, swivel-mounted on a grave and activated by trip wires.[15]

In her remarkable biography of John Hunter, *The Surgeon's Knife,* Wendy Moore describes many accounts of his dealings with resurrectionists to supply his brother's amphitheater with a steady flow of dissecting material, which were then beautifully immortalized by the renowned medical illustrator Jan van Rymsdyk (Fig. 35).[16] For the purpose of their didactic dissections, the brothers Hunter relied mostly on these shady procurements. For his scientific endeavors, John was particularly interested in specific human pathology, and could be even more proactive in procuring a specimen. One of his most famous "specimens" was the body of Charles Byrne, the "Irish giant." Byrne suffered from what we now know was acromegaly, an anomaly of the pituitary gland (in his case because of a tumor) that causes excess secretion of growth hormone. Although Byrne explicitly did not want his body dissected after his death (he had already been pursued by other anatomists), it was stolen by Hunter, who added the giant's skeleton to his collection.[17] The skeleton is still on display at the Royal College of Surgeons in London as part of the Hunterian Collection, which is why his underlying disease could be confirmed: the growing tumor in the pituitary gland, of course long gone, had eroded the sella turcica, the bony structure that cradles the gland, the hallmark of acromegaly.

Grave robbery was an all too common source of bodies for eighteenth- and nineteenth-century anatomists, but there is no proof that their creative requisitioning generally went any further. Still, there were rumors, and in a few well-publicized cases, there was hard evidence. The most notorious of these extreme body snatchers—who resorted to killing people, rather than waiting for them to die a natural death—were William Burke and William Hare.[18] Both criminals helped Dr. Robert Knox, a Scottish surgeon, obtain specimens for his anatomy courses at Surgeon's Square in Edinburgh. Knox himself was never charged, but Burke and Hare were; Hare eventually betrayed his acolyte in return for a lenient sentence. Burke was executed and his body was, ironically, used for an anatomic dissection, and his skin used as a pocketbook cover. His name lives on—pejoratively: *burking* is an English expression meaning to kill by suffocation or, figuratively, to stifle, conceal, or suppress.

The laws that restricted the use of cadavers for the purpose of anatomic research to the bodies of criminals were clearly meant to protect law-abiding members of society. However, the rising interest in medical education and its increasing demand for dissectible bodies—along with a steady decrease in executions—ushered in the English Anatomy Act of 1832, which sanctioned the use of bodies that were unclaimed and even allowed for voluntary donation of one's body to science, provided no next of kin objected.[19] Several well-known surgeons of that era, among them Dr. Charles Bell (see chapter 2) lobbied for the law to be passed, and the series of murders by Burke and Hare helped sway public opinion.

This law, like similar ones in other countries, still fall short of our modern understanding of autonomy and informed consent. Today, anatomic dissections in Western medical schools rely solely on cadavers that have been voluntarily bequeathed and no longer on unclaimed bodies. Research on human subjects (and, by extension, the utilization of human subjects, alive or dead, for the purpose of education) is strictly codified by the 1975 Declaration of Helsinki. The Declaration followed the Nuremberg Medical Trials after World War II, and led in the United States to the creation of the National Commission for the Protection of Human Subjects of Biomedical and Behavioral Research. That commission issued the Belmont report in 1978, which outlined three basic ethical principles: Respect for persons, beneficence, and justice.[20] Respect for persons includes the right to autonomy: with very few exceptions, a person must be able to grant consent, freely and without coercion, to participate in a research study or, in the case of anatomic dissection, to donate his or her body to science. Clearly, that would exclude the bodies of executed criminals, and it also protects prisoners from giving their consent, as they cannot do so freely.

A Tainted Beauty

Today's ethical norms guide our behavior in scientific and medical research, and we look back at the excesses of history with some air of superiority. We cannot morally separate ourselves from the past, however, even in so theoretical a discipline as medical illustration. Nowhere is this more evident than with the Pernkopf atlas—one of history's greatest anatomic reference books. Eduard Pernkopf was an Austrian professor of anatomy, department chair, and later rector at the University of Vienna. In 1933, he started to work on his *Topographische Anatomie des Menschen* (Human topographic anatomy) in collaboration with several medical illustrators. The work would become the most detailed and beautifully illustrated atlas of anatomy of its time, and is still considered a masterwork today. In that same year (1933), he joined the National Socialist (Nazi) Party, as did at least three of his artist collaborators, Erich Lepier, Karl Endtresser and Franz Batke. More than a mere Nazi sympathizer, Pernkopf became an active participant, purging the university of any Jewish faculty and actively promoting racial purity.[21]

Pernkopf himself was in a position of immense power at the University of Vienna, and his active participation in the horrors of the Nazi regime is undeniable. Can the same be said about his collaborators? Collectively, the Germans and Austrians allowed these atrocities to occur, but active opposition took more than principle: resistance could be a life-threatening decision, so most chose to go along. After the war, many "collaborators" of the Nazi regime were outed, but they had often done so out of passive cowardice, rather than as an active choice. The artists who illustrated the Pernkopf atlas, however, proudly advertised their allegiance. Karl Endtresser signed his name using the runic form for the double S in his name, referring to the Schutzstaffel (or SS) troops. Similarly, Franz Batke turned the 44 (for 1944) in his dated signatures into the SS sign. Erich Lepier added a swastika to the end of his name in his signature. These Nazi references were erased in later editions, although traces persisted for a while (Fig. 100).[22]

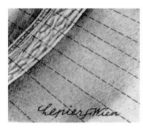

Fig. 100: Erich Lepier's signature in Pernkopf's atlas between 1941 and 1943. The swastika after his name was erased in later editions of the atlas.

History is rife with examples of unsavory characters who created artistic masterpieces, shattered athletic records, or made landmark scientific discoveries. Alexis Carrel was a French surgeon who received the Nobel Prize in physiology or medicine in 1912 for the development of vascular anastomosis. With Charles Lindbergh, he also developed a perfusion pump to allow organs to remain viable outside the body. Both endeavors paved the way for organ transplantation, making Carrel one of the pillars of this brand-new field in medicine. Carrel was also a fierce defender of eugenics,[23] as was Lindbergh, who openly advocated for the supremacy of the white race. Marcel Proust, author of *A la recherche du temps perdu* (Remembrances of things past), professed similar views. In more recent times, Roman Polanski's films and Michael Jackson's or R. Kelly's music have been widely praised by critics and the public alike, while their characters and actions have been justifiably vilified. How we choose to separate art or achievement from their author is a matter of personal choice and a topic of strong controversy. Should we handle the Nazi past of the world's most gifted medical illustrators differently?

The anatomic plates in the Pernkopf atlas are remarkable for their beauty, as well as their accuracy. The details of the vascular and nerve anatomy are found nowhere else; they are based on the direct observation of painstaking anatomic dissections to a level of complexity that had not been seen before. The plates are works of art as well. Eduard Pernkopf's explicit instructions had been to add color in such a way that the tissues would look "alive," while color-coding the various structures for easy recognition: the nerves are of an unnatural yellow, the arteries red, and the veins blue, but the full picture looks completely natural.[24] Surface rendering is so perfect that the epiploic fat on the sigmoid colon appears appropriately moist and glistening, the adrenal gland is lobulated and soft in consistency, the kidneys tense yet elastic inside their capsule. The Pernkopf atlas is a masterpiece, precisely because it is beautiful and accurate—the epitome of medical illustration.[25]

Should we separate the art (or science) from the author, no matter how monstrous his or her character? In the case of medical illustration, it is not just about the moral fiber of the artist. With regard to the Pernkopf atlas, the personal lives of its author and illustrators call into question the provenance of their material. Following an article by Howard Israel and William Seidelman in the *Journal of the American Medical Association* (*JAMA*) and a piece in the *New York Times* in 1996, an investigation was launched into the origin of the anatomic preparations used for the Pernkopf illustrations.[26] The University of Vienna created a historical research committee, the Senatorial Project.[27] It was financially supported, in part, by Edward B. Hutton, the president of Waverly, Inc. (Waverly had bought the original publishing house of the atlas, Urban & Schwarzenberg, the preceding year.) The committee found that between 1938 and 1945, the University of Vienna received almost four thousand unclaimed adult bodies for use in the anatomy laboratory, as well as thousands of fetuses, stillborn babies, and children who had died from natural causes. They also received more than thirteen hundred bodies of executed people. Very few of these victims were Jewish, the commission concluded, but there is no question that many of the executions would have been politically motivated.[28] Contrary to what was feared, there was no clear evidence that bodies from nearby concentration camps were brought to the University of Vienna. However, Herwig Czech and Erich Brenner, in a 2018 article in *Annals of Anatomy,* confirmed that histological specimens derived from Nazi victims were used for student examinations at the universities of Innsbruck and Graz as late as 1980.[29]

In the end, "only" forty-one plates from the Pernkopf atlas have been confirmed to be from executed prisoners, while the provenance of many others remains unclear. The atlas itself is no longer in print, but a large number of copies remain. Since August 1997, the rector's office of the University of Vienna has provided all libraries with an insert that states: "Currently, it cannot be excluded that certain preparations used for the illustrations in this atlas were obtained from (political) victims of the National Socialist regime. Furthermore, it is unclear whether cadavers were at that time supplied to the Institute of Anatomy at the University of Vienna not only from the Vienna district court but also from concentration camps. Pending the results of the investigation, it is therefore within the individual user's ethical responsibility to decide whether and in which way he wishes to use this book."[30]

The ethical dilemma surrounding the origins and the use of the Pernkopf atlas have generated a much more heated debate than older works with equally shady pasts. As D. Gareth Jones put it, "the history of anatomy is one of scientific knowledge gained at the 'edge of cultures,' sometimes transgressing the edge into the territory of crime and atrocities."[31] One explanation is the intricate relationship between the Nazi horrors and the emergence of our modern code of ethics regarding medical research on human subjects.

With the Declaration of Helsinki in 1975, the World Medical Association designed a code of conduct regarding human research, which states: "Reports on experimentation not in accordance with the principles laid down in this Declaration should not be accepted for publication."[32] In the United States, this was followed by the Belmont report, which referred to other blatant violations against humanity.[33] One such example is the government-sanctioned Tuskegee Airmen trial. In that longitudinal study, members of this all-black elite Air Force squadron who were diagnosed with syphilis were randomized without their knowledge into either a treatment arm or a placebo arm to observe the natural progression of the disease. The Tuskegee Airmen tragedy and other violations of human rights eventually led to the creation of Institutional Review Boards (IRB). These ethics committees operate independently in hospitals, medical schools, and other institutions where human research is conducted, but they answer to strict federal laws and regulations, the so-called "Common Rule," to ensure that research is scientifically sound and respectful of its human subjects. Regulations extend to research on deceased subjects, and therefore includes anatomic research as well.

How, then, should the tainted Pernkopf atlas be used? Simply rejecting it would be morally straightforward, but probably too simplistic.[34] Garrett Riggs asks whether "a creative or scientific work can be regarded as beautiful even if it was conceived in evil and born of malevolence?"[35] In other words, should the quality of the work even be considered?[36] Most scholars agree that bad science should be rejected, and that any information obtained from scientifically flawed experiments should be denounced. An often-cited example is the hypothermia experiments conducted by Nazi doctors in concentration camps, whereby prisoners were subjected to a lethal level of cold exposure, often without anesthesia, to examine the body's responses.[37] Beyond the cruelty of these so-called experiments, any scientific merit has since been debunked. It is therefore obvious that the results of these experiments should never be accepted or used. There is a distinction, however, between flawed scientific research, like the hypothermia experiments, "sound" scientific research obtained through coercion, and research on already deceased bodies, as is the case with the Pernkopf atlas. It is undeniable that the quality of that atlas is unsurpassed. In a fascinating article, Andrew Yee describes a rare case of saphenous nerve entrapment whereby the anatomy of a patient was so unusual that only the Pernkopf atlas gave the surgeon enough detail to successfully complete the operation and provide relief for the patient where prior interventions had failed.[38] None of the other anatomic atlases, such as Henry Gray's and Frank Netter's, had been detailed enough to be of use in that particular instance.

If one has access to a copy of the atlas, should he or she be justified in consulting it? Ethically, the short answer may still be *no*. We should not encourage illicit or morally reprehensible behavior by publicizing or using its results, an argument that is also being used increasingly by responsible media outlets when they refuse to name mass killers and other criminals, and give a voice to their victims instead.[39] But if the work already exists, why could the images not be used? After all, they are several times removed from the original unethical act: even though the human subjects may have been used illicitly, this concerns color reproductions of paintings made of already deceased people. Utilizing copies of existing anatomic plates is unlikely to create a greater demand for illicit human dissections. Some religious scholars would even argue that, if it can save a life, it is not only justifiable but mandatory to use any scientifically sound research material.[40] Some, like Sabine Hildebrandt, scientific researcher and associate professor of pediatrics at Harvard Medical School, have pointed out that using these anatomic plates, with due expression of respect for their victims, is a way to go against the Nazi plans to forever silence classes of human beings—Jews, as well as Romas, people with disabilities, and others they considered inferior. Michel Atlas (yes, that is his real name) argues that "it is ironic retribution for the Jewish cadavers (or whoever died for whatever their beliefs) used to illustrate a Nazi's anatomic atlas to be immortalized by it. Using this atlas allows these cadavers to speak to us from half a century ago. They make us reexamine and again repudiate the Nazi beliefs that created a society that killed them."[41] In other words, using the atlas would glorify and immortalize the very people the Nazis tried to exterminate. They are rehabilitated through their paintings.[42]

Other authors, like Riggs and Richard Panush, argue that this atlas can easily be replaced by other works, and that equally detailed atlases of human anatomy exist.[43] An example cited by Riggs is the Sobotta atlas, which has been in press for almost a century, and is used by countless medical schools, mostly in Europe. Johannes Sobotta published the first edition of his book in 1904, more than three decades before the rise of the Nazi regime, and therefore theoretically beyond reproach. However, later editions of Sobotta's atlas have incorporated many plates by Lepier and Endtresser, of Pernkopf fame.[44] Should Sobotta's books be banned? Or just the plates in question? The addition of illustrations by Pernkopf's artists occurred after the war and before the controversy came to light. This exonerates the atlas from accusations of utilizing victims of war atrocities as their subjects, but not of its collaborators' Nazi past. Another solution is to move away from illustrated anatomy atlases altogether now that modern imaging technology affords us an even better view at the macroscopic and microscopic anatomy of humans. The most notorious example—and one that is cited by Sabine Hildebrandt—is the Visible Human Project, sponsored by the National Institutes of Health.[45] This ambitious undertaking was made possible by someone who donated his body after his death. It consisted of a whole-body computerized axial tomography (CT) scan, followed by millimeter-thick axial slicing of the preserved body to allow correlation of radiologic and pathologic images. Using computer-enhanced volume rendering of the slices, a complete, detailed, fully searchable 3-D atlas of human anatomy was produced. Yet this project attracted its own controversy: the "volunteer" who gave his body to science was a prisoner on death row. While he may have given consent for the procedure, the Belmont report clearly states that prisoners and other nonautonomous individuals can never consent of their own free will, and while there are exceptions to the ban on studies on prisoners, this project did not reach the high bar placed on such research.[46] It is quite an interesting coda to the story of how, for centuries, the discovery and illustration of human anatomy occurred through the dissection of criminals, a practice that had been universally abandoned in modern times.

Medical illustration, and the study of anatomy specifically, may have a shady past, but outright crimes and gross ethical abuses are now history. That doesn't mean that its current record is spotless. In many circles, professions, and disciplines, the existence of implicit bias, unequal treatment based on gender or race, and other social disparities are being increasingly recognized and addressed. The field of medical illustration is not immune to that long-overdue movement, and some reflection is taking place.

Take Frank Netter and his vivid illustrations showing the manifestations of Cushing's syndrome, hypertension, emphysema, and other common diseases (see Fig. 1). Frank Netter has had his detractors, mostly purists who feel that he compromised scientific and anatomic accuracy in favor of esthetics, and they definitely have a point. But his descriptions of medical "tableaux" are what sets him apart from the anatomists who came before him. He may not be the first or the only one to depict the human body in such a naturalistic way, but he can be rightfully credited with helping generations of medical, nursing, and medical illustration students understand anatomy, pathophysiology, pathology, and all manner of surgery. His illustrations have a distinct 1950s feel, and are quintessentially American. The comparison with Norman Rockwell is inescapable.[47] (Rockwell and Netter were friends, and both were disciples of the "Ashcan School" movement in American art, so called for its emphasis on daily life scenes.)

However, nostalgia should not stand in the way of some self-analysis. Netter's paintings, like Rockwell's, are folksy depictions of 1950s life in America, which—if one believes the *Saturday Evening Post* covers—was mostly white middle class, a very homogeneous society with very few black and brown people, and—ironically, for illustrations of medical conditions—no people with disabilities. While modern society now sees this lack of diversity in popular representation as a thing of the past, the field of medical illustration may have been slow to adapt. What's more, this lack of diverse iconography has helped perpetuate the "old ways" and hindered inclusion. In an enlightened interview, Jill Gregory, a certified medical illustrator and associate director of the Instructional Technology Group at the Icahn School of Medicine in New York, describes this problem with vivid examples.[48] In an attempt to come across as clean, sterile, and nonthreatening, many illustrations of someone having a heart attack or a blockage of coronary arteries (especially in ads for pharmaceutical companies) show a generic thirtysomething male clutching his chest, with a glowing red heart projected through his thorax to indicate the source of the pain. Why does it have to be a young man when myocardial infarction is most common in people in their sixties or seventies? A recent article on a shocking statistic—that puerperal mortality (mothers dying in childbirth) is still unacceptably high in the United States at twenty-four out of one hundred thousand births—was illustrated with a photograph of a white woman cuddling a newborn baby even though the most shocking part of the study was that African American mothers were three to four times more likely to die in childbirth than white mothers. People of color are disproportionally at risk for many diseases, including diabetes and hypertension, yet they are underrepresented in medical illustrations, as are the elderly, people with disabilities, and women. What harm can this do, one might ask, as long as the research and information is accurate? After all, these are only illustrations. However, being unable to recognize oneself in images can lead to marginalization and a feeling of not being represented. It can also be hazardous to your health: depiction of common dermatological conditions, for example, is too often based on appearance in white-skinned individuals. Rashes, moles, and melanoma can look very different in dark-skinned individuals, and many have recently decried a lack of diversity in dermatology textbooks and medical school lectures.[49]

Much has been said about the distrust some segments of the population have toward the scientific and medical community. With the COVID-19 pandemic, vaccine hesitancy in black and brown people has been a common media trope, often illustrated by that other trope, the previously mentioned Tuskegee Airmen syphilis study.[50] The reason for distrust of medical authorities is clearly much more complex than a single historic event, and (re)gaining that trust has to start with inclusion and representation—and medical illustration certainly has a role to play in this.

It may be commendable to try and make an illustration as generic as possible, in order to make it relatable to a large audience. Showing too many identifying characteristics about a model makes the example more unique and therefore less applicable to the general population. A recent trend has been to make characters in pharmaceutical and medical imagery generically blue-skinned to make them race- or even gender-neutral. (The blue color of the model also contrasts nicely with a typically "red-hot" aching body part, particularly in ads and commercials for joint pain relief.) This results in esthetically pleasing, but sanitized, inoffensive designs that avoid confronting anatomical, racial, age, and gender diversity. There is a legitimate concern, however, that averaging the representation of a human being diminishes us all. It has also been noted that these "generic" characters clearly have Caucasian features. This whole exercise has been derisively called "blue white guy."[51]

Medical illustrations are the face of medicine—in ads and commercials, in textbooks, in scientific papers, on posters in doctors' offices, in official pamphlets from the Centers for Disease Control and Prevention (CDC) or the National Institutes of Health (NIH). Medical illustrators, therefore, have a social responsibility to reflect real life and real people.

Chapter 4

The Bright Side of Medical Illustration

For all the shady aspects of anatomic and medical illustration through the centuries, illustrators are far more often responsible for great discoveries and advances in medicine. As the Association of Medical Illustrators puts it, scientific illustrators are visual problem solvers. Their task is to analyze a concept, an operation, a pathophysiologic problem, the better to depict it in the most accurate and clear way. This requires more than just artistic talent: it assumes that the illustrator understands the problem at hand—either based on his or her own scientific background, or through collaboration with clinicians, researchers, or other scientists. Naturally, the line separating clinicians from illustrators is sometimes blurred, and examples abound where important medical and scientific discoveries were made in collaboration with, and sometimes led by illustrators.

Anatomic Discoveries

Max Brödel, the "fifth doctor" at the Johns Hopkins University Hospital in the late nineteenth century, was not only a gifted artist but a very dedicated and meticulous one as well. He believed in depicting exactly what was there without embellishments or shortcuts. Whether it was an anatomical illustration or the figure for a surgical atlas, he was known to research the topic thoroughly, exactly like a scientific researcher would proceed. Upon his arrival in Baltimore, he worked closely with Howard Kelly, the chief of obstetrics and gynecology,

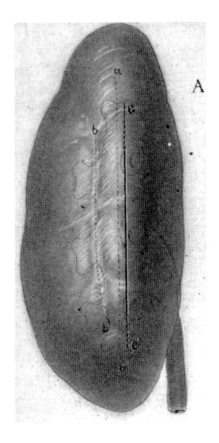

Fig. 101: Max Brödel, Plate XXXV: Lateral aspect of left kidney, showing the location of the most advantageous incision through the parenchyma in kidneys, which have a normal arterial arrangement, in *The Intrinsic Blood-Vessels of the Kidney and Their Significance in Nephrotomy,* Proceedings of the Association of American Anatomists, 1900. A duplicative paler area of the kidney's capsule, adjacent to the posterior midline, represents a relatively bloodless access to the renal parenchyma. This anatomic landmark is now known as the "white line of Brödel."

who needed Brödel's talents to illustrate his seminal textbooks on abdominal surgery, gynecological disorders, and diseases of the kidneys, ureters, and bladder. This required Brödel to spend countless hours in the operating room, observing Kelly as he performed the procedures that would ultimately be described in his atlases. Max Brödel's meticulous study of his subject also led to an important clinical discovery. Long before lithotripsy (ultrasonic pulverization) or endoscopic techniques were available to break down or remove kidney stones, the only option was surgical extirpation. This required not only an abdominal operation, but opening of the kidney as well. Kidneys are solid organs that are extremely well vascularized (they are fed by the renal arteries, which come directly off the aorta). The traditional approach to the renal pelvis, where the large stones were stuck, unable to pass down the ureter, was to randomly cut through the parenchyma of the kidney, leading to significant blood loss. Through repeated examination of these organs, Brödel noted that the blood supply to the anterior and posterior portions of the kidney met in the middle, and that a relatively blood vessel–free space existed in a plane immediately posterior to the coronal plane of the kidney, where the diameter of the vessels from both sides were at their smallest.[1] To the careful observer, that area appears paler because of the relative paucity of blood vessels, and if one opened the kidney along that line, blood loss could be much reduced. This anatomic landmark of the kidney is now known as the "white line of Brödel" (Fig. 101).

Brödel contributed to advancing medical knowledge in many ways during his tenure at Johns Hopkins Hospital, either alone or in association with the likes of Howard Kelly, Thomas Cullen and Edward Richardson (two other respected gynecologists),[2] William Halsted, the neurosurgeon Harvey Cushing, and others. Two telling examples are a monograph about the musculature of the anterior abdominal wall that started as an article by Thomas Cullen about hemorrhage into the rectus abdominis muscle,[3] and a book on the anatomy of the belly button. For both, Brödel was asked to do several illustrations, but ended up delving into the topics so thoroughly that Cullen insisted on giving him research credit. In his words, "I asked Mr. Brödel if he would make a few drawings graphically illustrating the gradual development of the umbilical region. After gaining a clear insight into the various abnormalities found in this region, he became most enthusiastic and undertook a thorough study of the subject. . . . I want to emphasize the fact that, although I wrote this chapter, the credit for the original research connected with the development of the accompanying drawings belongs entirely to Mr. Brödel."[4] In a move that seems to emulate da Vinci by cutting out the middleman, the medical illustrator became the scientist. Ever since Vesalius, researchers partnered with famous artists of their time to illustrate their anatomic discoveries. Some, like Max Brödel, could be both artist and scientist, emphasizing qualities shared by both professions: detailed observation and objectivity, and the skill to report exactly what is there without prejudice or preconceived ideas. Through the generosity of his medical colleagues, Max Brödel has received credit for many other contributions to anatomy research, including a chapter on the anatomy of the kidney in Howard Kelly's *Diseases of the Kidneys, Ureters and Bladder* and a chapter on the anatomy of the appendix in Kelly's "The Vermiform Appendix and Its Diseases."

Illustrators as Researchers

The development of a revolutionary operation by Patrick C. Walsh in the last decades of the twentieth century owes a lot to his collaboration with medical illustrator Leon Schlossberg. In the 1970s, radical prostatectomy significantly improved survival in men with prostate cancer. Unfortunately, the operation was fraught with the real risk of life-threatening hemorrhage and devastating side effects: 100 percent of patients became impotent postoperatively, and up to a quarter of them were incontinent. The treatment was perceived by doctors and patients as being worse than the disease,[5] and it was mostly abandoned in favor of less curative treatment modalities, such as external beam radiation. Dr. Walsh's major contribution was a painstaking study of the neurovascular anatomy around the prostate, which eventually led to a nerve-sparing technique that completely changed the treatment and outcome of prostate cancer. In Walsh's words, "Leon Schlossberg was more than a medical illustrator—he was an anatomist. By having him watch the operations and discuss the findings, we were able to develop a detailed understanding of the anatomy surrounding the prostate and identified minor anatomical details that were important to perfecting the surgical technique."[6]

Many other medical illustrators have thus blurred the lines between research and didactics, and can be rightfully included in the scientific teams they represent. In 1943, Ranice W. Crosby was the first woman to head the Department of Arts as Applied to Medicine—and the first woman heading *any* department at the Johns Hopkins School of Medicine. She is credited, alongside Elizabeth Ramsey, with the understanding of placental physiology (Fig. 102).[7] Dorcas Hager Padget, another member of the Hopkins team, worked for years with the neurosurgeon Walter Dandy, and illustrated many of his publications. Detailed observation of the subjects she was asked to illustrate led to

Fig. 102: Ranice W. Crosby, Structure, physiology, and circulation of the placenta in higher primates, in Elizabeth M. Ramsey, *The Placenta: Human and Animal.* (Courtesy of the Carnegie Institution for Science.)

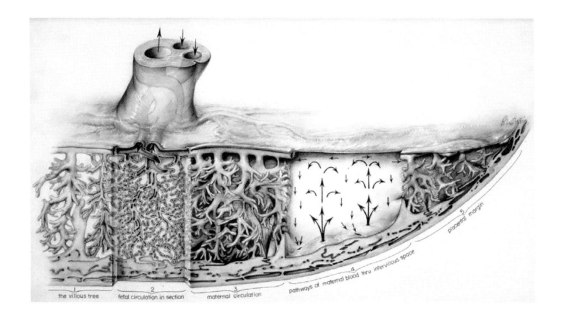

further research in normal and abnormal neurovascular physiology and anatomy. Dandy's textbook on intracranial aneurysms, titled *The Circle of Willis: Its Embryology and Anatomy,* contains a chapter that was not only illustrated but written by Padget.[8] With encouragement from Dandy, she conducted research on the embryology of the blood vessels of the brain using the Carnegie Collection of human embryos, and published many papers and monographs on the vascular anatomy of the brain. In addition to being a gifted illustrator, she was an especially effective one: her work is touted as a gold standard for effective medical "storytelling."[9] Dorcas Padget is rightfully remembered as an embryologist, a scientist in her own right.[10] She is generally cocredited with clarifying the development of two neuropathological phenomena, the Arnold-Chiari malformation, and the Dandy-Walker syndrome.[11]

When medical illustrators first became essential members of a medical research team, gross human anatomy was in its infancy. Illustrators observed anatomists as they dissected cadavers and dutifully reproduced their findings. In the ensuing centuries, macroscopic anatomy no longer held many secrets for physicians and students. While illustrators continued to offer their work to institutions of higher learning, the discovery phase was mostly over, save for the very occasional reporting of a never-before recognized anatomic structure. (In 2016, a Swiss team led by Karl Grob published the discovery of a "new" muscle in the leg, the tensor of the vastus intermedius.[12] In 2020, a Dutch group "discovered" a hitherto unknown salivary gland.[13]) The introduction of the microscope, followed by centuries of technical advances, shifted the field of anatomy to the microscopic—down to cellular and subcellular anatomy. In Vesalius's time, the task of the medical illustrator had been to make the findings of gross anatomic dissection accessible to all to help disseminate medical knowledge. As scientists started to study the unseen, the function of illustrators changed. Rather than report what everyone could see, they had to interpret what was not visible to the naked eye, translating what researchers could only discern using specialized instruments. Antonie Van Leeuwenhoek is generally credited as the inventor of the microscope in the late seventeenth century. As he was discovering structures that had never been seen before, he was forced to use analogies for artists to reproduce what he saw. In examining muscle fibers under the microscope, he described "[fibers that] looked like so many boughs of trees, with the leaves on them," an image that was dutifully reproduced by an artist in the Philosophical Transactions of the Royal Society, of which Van Leeuwenhoek was a member (Fig. 103).[14] Robert Hooke, a contemporary and colleague of Van Leeuwenhoek, is credited with the

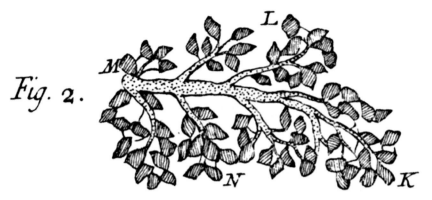

Fig. 103: Carnous fibers, in Antonie Van Leeuwenhoek, *Philosophical Transactions*, 1720, vol. 31, p. 131.

first description of cells, and coining that term. Examining thin slices of cork oak under the microscope, the honeycomb appearance of dead bark reminded him of rows of small rooms in a monastery, called cells (from the Latin *cella* [storeroom], which also gave us *cellar*).

To Infinitely Small and Beyond

As people discovered ever smaller structures, it became increasingly important to describe and explain these findings in terms that others would easily understand: from monastic cells to branches and leaves on a tree to trees themselves: three centuries later, a team of medical illustrators helped make a significant discovery in the structure and function of dendritic cells. Dendritic cells (from the Greek *dendros* [tree]) are cells that were identified decades ago as antigen-presenting cells (APC). An essential part of the immune system, they somehow get foreign particles, like bacterial or viral material, to attach themselves to the treelike excrescences on their cell membrane (Fig. 104). This facilitates the engulfment and destruction of the antigen by a T-lymphocyte, a specialized white blood cell that will also recognize the antigen in the future, an essential step in acquired immunity. The synergy between the APC and the T-cell had been recognized for a long time, but the exact mechanism by which the dendritic cell was able to attract and retain the antigens long enough to be destroyed by a T-cell was unknown. Collaboration between cellular scientists and medical illustrators led to the recognition that what appear as dendrites or filopodia (threadlike filaments) in two dimensions are in fact wavy sheets or folds of cell membrane that trap particles in their recesses (Fig. 105).[15] Similar discoveries have been made about other cells and cell organelles by analyzing the two-dimensional data of transmission electron microscopy (EM), and extrapolating information from three-

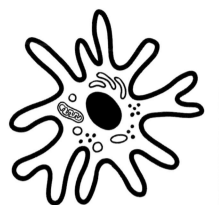

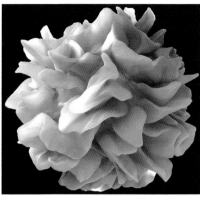

dimensional scanning EM images. It took visual artists to reconcile the various cross sections to what we now believe are the true volumetric shapes of these microscopic structures. Beyond the creation of "pretty pictures" to help popularize scientific discoveries, medical illustrators are full-fledged members of the research teams, using their skills to explain cellular and subcellular anatomy.

Sometimes the medical illustrator is the only one who can see the full picture, and holds the key to a problem that has not otherwise been fully solved. In an opinion piece in *Scientific American,* Veronica Falconieri Hays deconstructs the visualization of the SARS-CoV-2 coronavirus, source of the COVID-19 pandemic.[16] As she puts it, building a workable 3-D model of the complete virus "required a mix of research, hypothesis and artistic license." While much was already known about some of the components of the novel virus, this information was gathered from research on other, similar coronaviruses. The overall shape and size of the virion were known, as was the rough shape of the spike proteins (S) that stud the organism's outer core and give it its name (corona, or crown). However, some of the S protein's parts, like the stem and the tail, are flexible and constantly morphing, and had eluded our understanding of what they look like in real life. (Looking for known analogies, Falconieri Hays refers to the first pass at illustrating the spikes as "rock candy lollipops.") The ultimate result became a three-dimensional model that was a combination of known structures, best guesses based on other, similar particles, and deductions from functional studies on the virus's interactions with host cells. No longer is the medical illustrator a "scribe" who reports on the work of scientists. She is a scientist herself, gathering detailed, specialized information from various laboratories and myriad diagnostic techniques, even collaborating with research colleagues and networking on "science Twitter."[17]

Medical illustrators have thus helped us understand the spatial configuration of cells and organelles that can be seen only through highly specialized instruments, utilizing a visual language that we can all relate to: that of the macroscopic world (trees, branches, lollipops). But what about structures that are even smaller than that—structures that can't be seen at all, not even with the most powerful instrument? At the molecular level, it's all about atoms, nuclei, and electrons. Most middle-schoolers have had to create a 3-D model of a molecule, typically represented by several Styrofoam spheres connected by rods, each atom color-coded to literally reflect the molecule's composition: a black ball for carbon, a white one for each of the two hydrogen atoms and three gray oxygen atoms: there's your carbonic acid molecule (Fig. 106). This is not what these molecules look like in the wild, of course, and it is only slightly more didactic than the written formula (H_2CO_3). Whereas carbonic acid, hydrogen sulfate, glucose ($C_6H_{12}O_6$), or any of the amino acids are relatively easy to

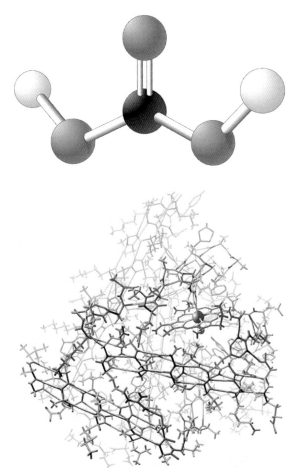

Fig. 106: *Top:* Graphic representation of a molecule of carbonic acid: one central carbon atom (black), two hydrogen atoms (white), and three oxygen atoms (gray). *Bottom:* Irving Geis, *Myoglobin,* 1961. Molecular structure of the myoglobin molecule of the sperm whale. In Martin Kemp's words, "Geis [used] his unrivalled command of perspective, light and shade, and [color] recession to reveal the intricate sculptural web of linkages." (Martin Kemp, "Kendrew Constructs; Geis Gazes," *Nature* 396, no. 6711 (1998): 525, https://doi.org/10.1038/25019. Image from the Irving Geis Collection, Howard Hughes Medical Institute (HHMI). Rights owned by HHMI. Not to be used without permission.)

display that way, macromolecules are much more difficult to depict. Albumin, one of the most ubiquitous proteins, contains more than five hundred amino acids. Collagen has more than one thousand and myosin more than two thousand.

The graphic representation of such complex structures requires the creative talent to assemble the atoms and molecules correctly while simultaneously showing a cohesive, recognizable, and reproducible three-dimensional object. Irving Geis was an artist and illustrator who collaborated closely with biologists, and a pioneer in the depiction of macromolecules. His illustration of myoglobin in a 1961 article in *Scientific American* is a remarkable example of the role of a medical illustrator: to clearly explain a complex and sometimes abstract concept (Fig. 106).[18] Myoglobin is a 154-amino acid macromolecule that is related to hemoglobin. It is abundantly present in skeletal and heart muscle cells. Its clinical relevance lies in its detection in blood and urine when there is significant muscle trauma and disruption, as with crush injuries and myocardial infarction. The crystal structure of myoglobin was discovered by John Kendrew in 1958, using X-ray crystallography. (Kendrew, together with Max Perutz, was awarded the Nobel Prize in chemistry for that discovery.) It was Geis's representation of the complex three-dimensional relationships between the amino acids, the ferrous heme ring, and its oxygen bond that allowed other scientists to understand the function of this and many other macromolecules.

In Geis's model of myoglobin, each amino acid is represented by a distinct stick figure, and the resulting three-dimensional volume resembles a wild Meccano Erector set. It is a clear representation of the relationship of amino acids in space, but it is still too simplistic to reflect the real-life shape of biologic building blocks. The primary bonds between any two molecules are what strings a macromolecule together, but the higher order bonds that occur naturally between adjacent sections of a macromolecule dictate its overall three-dimensional shape. A single molecule substitution can alter the bond between two distant portions of a macromolecule, thereby totally reshaping its ultrastructure or its relationship to other molecules.

A well-known example of how a single difference in amino acid sequence can alter the function of a protein is hemoglobin S, the cause of sickle-cell anemia. Hemoglobin is a protein that is essential to the transport of oxygen in the blood. Because oxygen is not water-soluble, it must be actively bound to a "carrier" molecule to be absorbed from the air we breathe and transported to all the cells in our body, where the carrier molecule releases the oxygen molecules. Hemoglobin, the

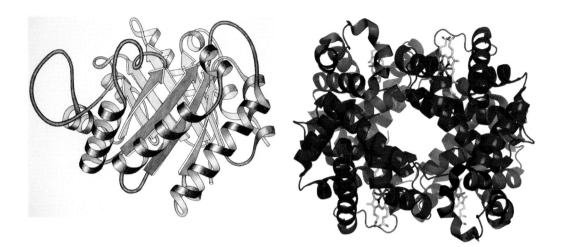

carrier molecule, is abundant in red blood cells. Its basic structure is composed of four separate units of 141 amino acids each—two α chains and two β chains, each containing a heme ring that binds one oxygen molecule (Fig. 107).

The sequence of the first thirty amino acids in the β-globin is *val-his-leu-thr-pro-**glu**-glu-lys-ser-ala-val-thr-ala-leu-trp-gly-lys-val-asn-val-asp-glu-val-gly-gly-glu-ala-leu-gly-arg* (where each three-letter code stands for one of the twenty-two amino acids found in nature: *val* = valine, *glu* = glutamate, *trp* = tryptophan, and so on). For geneticists, this is a very helpful representation. Sickle-cell anemia is caused by a single nucleotide mutation in a gene on the short arm of chromosome 11, which results in the abnormal coding of a single amino acid in the β chain of hemoglobin: the glutamate molecule in the sixth position (underlined and bold in the above formula) is replaced by a molecule of valine. How does this single switch in amino acid lead to the full spectrum of symptoms that patients with sickle-cell anemia suffer? The answer is that instead of a water-soluble state in which each hemoglobin molecule floats around independently, the valine site of the abnormal β globin interacts with areas on adjacent hemoglobin molecules, particularly in low oxygen tension environments. This leads to molecular stacking—the assembly of multiple hemoglobin molecules in linear polymers that form filaments: long, rigid rods that span the width of a red blood cell and cause it to change shape.[19] Instead of a round, biconcave disc that is flexible and easily flows through even the narrowest of blood vessels, the cell turns into a rigid quarter moon—or sickle-shaped—structure that gets stuck and blocks the capillaries. As many of these tiny vessels are blocked, oxygen delivery to the downstream tissues is impaired, leading to all sorts of damage—infarcts, ischemia, and necrosis, which

Fig. 107: *Left:* Jane Richardson, hand-drawn and hand-colored "Ribbon" schematic of the protein triosephosphate isomerase, 1981. (Licensed under CC BY 3.0.) *Right:* Richard Wheeler (Zephyris), 2007, drawing of the hemoglobin tetramer molecule: 2 α globins, in red, and 2 β, globins, in blue, each with one heme ring (green) that binds with one oxygen molecule. (Licensed under CC Attribution-Share Alike 3.0.)

cause severe pain and can become a nidus for infections, such as osteomyelitis (infection of the bone) and pneumonia. These abnormal red blood cells also break down more rapidly than normal erythrocytes when they get stuck in tortuous arterioles and capillaries. Increased cell death leads to a paucity of red blood cells, or anemia, which affects overall well-being, increases fatigue, and causes cardiac strain as the heart must pump faster to deliver the same amount of oxygen to the tissues with a lower number of oxygen-carrying cells. Faster breakdown of red blood cells leads to an increased release of their content, including hemoglobin. Degradation of hemoglobin in the liver involves separation of the molecule into its four globin parts, recycling of the iron atoms, and breakdown of the heme rings into biliverdin, a pigment that is one of the components of bile. Excess red blood cell breakdown (hemolysis) leads to excessive concentrations of bile pigments in the bile, which causes it to sediment and form gallstones. This, in turn, can lead to acute cholecystitis (infection of the gallbladder), chronic calculous cholecystitis (abdominal pain caused by inflammation of the stones-filled gallbladder, especially after meals), choledocholithiasis (blockage of the bile ducts by a stone), cholangitis (severe infection of the bile ducts), and gallstone pancreatitis (acute inflammation of the adjacent pancreatic duct caused by the passage of a common bile duct stone).

Understanding the pathophysiology of sickle-cell anemia is both fascinating (a single DNA coding error leads to this vast spectrum of symptoms) and deceptively simple to understand. Depicting the structure of large proteins like hemoglobin is much more difficult. And yet, the three-dimensional representation of macromolecules is essential to understand the interaction between these structures as they regulate every single aspect of life. It is the three-dimensional structure of receptors that allows them to bind to specific signaling proteins and not to others, as elegantly demonstrated with the ultrastructure of the coronavirus. Furthermore, the interaction between a messenger and its receptor effectuates a change in the actual shape of the macromolecules that leads to the downstream activation of a pathway or the opening of a cellular channel, much like a mechanical switch. How, then, to portray the three-dimensional appearance of proteins and other macromolecules while remaining true to their basic chemical structure? This conceptual problem was solved by medical illustrators.

Jane Richardson is a professor of biochemistry at Duke University who, with her husband and fellow biochemist David, designed the ribbon diagram to depict the secondary and tertiary structures of proteins (Fig. 107).[20] Originally done in pencil and watercolor, they are still the most common method to describe the spatial relations of amino acids, carbohydrates, and other building blocks within complex molecules. Their perfection lies in the balance between the depiction of each individual base molecule (think valine and glutamate) and the overall image of the entire structure. It is not an abstract series of letters on a string, but neither is it a realistic microphotograph of a protein: it is an instructional tool that helps scientists visualize the shape of ultramicroscopic structures, and thereby understand their function in all aspects of life.[21] From the early drawings, an entire new vocabulary emerged: polypeptides can be folded upon themselves as "hairpins," rolled into alpha horseshoes, beta propellers, or jelly rolls. The seemingly naive drawings of ribbons and tubes are a translation of findings obtained by X-ray crystallography and other esoteric methods to identify macromolecules.

In fact, the most iconic image of a macromolecule owes its existence to X-ray crystallography. Rosalind Franklin and Raymond Gosling, one of her PhD students, had worked on the structure of deoxyribonucleic acid (DNA) and produced a series of X-ray diffraction images. It was the famed photo no. 51 that provided Francis Crick and James Watson with the proof of a double helix. Demonstrating once again the power of collaboration between scientist and illustrator, Francis Crick's rough sketch was translated into a crisp, clean drawing of the double-stranded helix by his wife, Odile (Fig. 108) That illustration made it into Watson

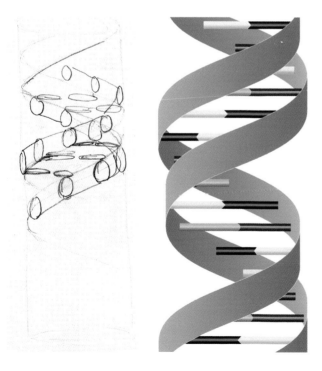

Fig. 108: The double-helix structure of DNA. *Left:* Francis Crick's rough sketch of the helix concept, based on Rosalind Franklin's X-ray diffraction photographs. (Wellcome Foundation, licensed under CC BY 4.0.0.) *Right:* Example of the iconic double-helix structure of DNA, originally created for Watson and Crick's landmark *Nature* paper by Odile Crick. (Licensed under CC BY 4.0.0.)

and Crick's landmark paper in *Nature* in 1953, and from there into the universal concept for all things genetic.[22] The marriage of art and science had a more personal and literal effect, too: Odile and Francis Crick's granddaughter, Kindra Crick, is a successful artist with a scientific background whose art is inspired by medicine and science.[23]

As we continue our journey of discovery into medicine and science, we realize that the spatial interaction between two large proteins, while complex, is still a simplistic way of understanding molecular biology. In reality, each type of immunoglobulin, enzyme receptor, antigen, and antibody has innumerable copies. All these structures interact with each other at the same time—as seen in the molecule-

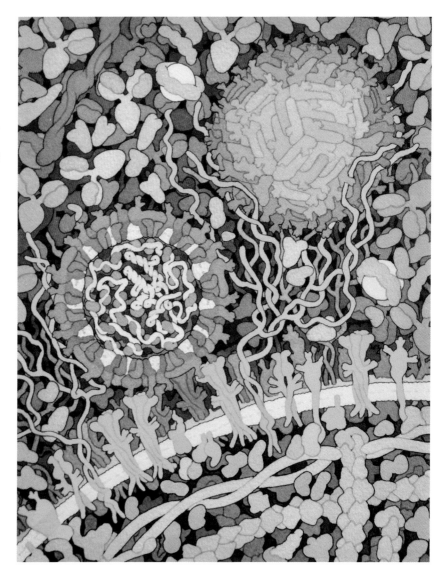

Fig. 109: The Zika virus, 2017. Illustration by David S. Goodsell, RCSB Protein Data Bank. https://doi.org/10.2210/rcsb_pdb/goodsell-gallery-015. (Licensed under CC BY 4.0.)

stacking example of sickle-cell anemia—and this entire soup of molecules is in constant flux, floating and colliding in the liquid intra- and extracellular environments.

It has become almost impossible to illustrate the cellular and ultrastructural reality with the classic tools of the illustrator. Fortunately, technology can help. David Goodsell, a structural biologist and professor of computational biology at the Scripps Research Institute, is credited for merging the art of illustration with the power of the computer to create three- and four-dimensional depictions of the activity inside a cell.[24] He and his colleagues created a Fortran computer program to create nonphotorealistic images of biological molecules.[25] (While he created the computer program to allow wide dissemination of images of macromolecules, his original depictions of intracellular life are painstakingly hand-painted watercolors.)

Here, too, the goal is not to obtain a realistic depiction of each molecule, each organelle, but rather to produce a comprehensible image of life under the electron microscope. His paintings become works of art, and each structure, each virion, each myofibril is designed to best reflect its size, shape, and function. It is also carefully colorized to make it immediately recognizable among the throngs of structures interacting in this microenvironment. In 2016, David Goodsell's painting of the Zika virus (Fig. 109) was recognized by the National Science Foundation (NSF) and *Popular Science* as one of the best science images of the year and selected as the "People's Choice" in the category of illustration.[26] Goodsell has updated his collection of "beautiful, but deadly" subjects with the 2020 release of a painting of the SARS-CoV-2 virus, responsible for the COVID-19 pandemic.[27] The addition of computerized animation makes it even more realistic, and has helped scientists better understand the individual interactions of proteins and other macromolecules on a global scale. More than ever, medical illustrators don't just visualize—they explain.

A Universal Language

Excellent visual artists have this in common with master clinicians: they are great observers of the world around us. They excel at looking without prejudice, discerning small details, seeing what is there rather than what they expect to see. Medical illustrators must possess these skills as well but just like clinicians, they use their talent of observation to advance medicine and science. They must therefore be great communicators. A good doctor must establish a bond with their patients, gain their trust, and explain in clear language what the diagnosis is, and what the treatment entails. Like any other profession, medicine has its own opaque jargon. In medicine, this includes impossibly long Latin words and arcane abbreviations (premature infants, for example, are at risk for necrotizing enterocolitis, retinopathy of prematurity, bronchopulmonary dysplasia, intraventricular hemorrhage, and persistent pulmonary hypertension of the neonate, or NEC, ROP, BPD, IVH, and PPHN, respectively). The scientific origin of diseases is based on increasingly complex concepts, and diagnostic and therapeutic methods are more and more technology driven. (Double spin-echo sequence rapid spectroscopic imaging of hyperpolarized ^{13}C, anyone?)

The doctor must communicate with the patient and the patient's family in ways that are simple yet accurate, straightforward without being patronizing. The language will be different when conversing with colleagues, and different still when teaching students and residents, the next generation of healers. Each audience has different needs and different expectations, and knowing one's audience is important.

Icons and Archetypes

The medical illustrator, like the clinician, must be a great communicator. Being a gifted artist is of course an asset, but medical illustration is not just about a pretty picture. The goal of a good scientific illustration is to communicate the essence of the subject, and to do it in the optimal way for the appropriate audience. This didactic calling is, of course, not unique to medical illustration. Before they were associated with anatomists, doctors, or scientists, many artists communicated with their audience, and needed ways to get their messages across. Classic examples abound in the graphic arts and are often rooted in religion. Religious symbolism may evoke mystic ideas, but often the goal was to appeal to the masses. In the days when an education was a privilege of the few and illiteracy was the norm, how could one depict religious concepts and stories in ways that the public could understand them? How, for example, could people distinguish one saint from another if they couldn't read their names? By identifying each character with

a particular attribute, itself a shortcut to a story attached to them. St. Peter, closest disciple of Christ and subject of the first pun in biblical history—"You are Petrus [stone], and on this stone, I will build my temple"— became associated with the gates of heaven, and as a gatekeeper, was always depicted with the keys to the heavenly kingdom (Fig. 110). St. John the Baptist, who lived an ascetic life in the wilderness, is usually depicted wearing an animal skin. Although he chose an austere lifestyle as an adult, he is depicted wearing an animal skin even as an infant or child. He is said to have been a childhood friend of Jesus, and when they are portrayed together, as in Michelangelo's *The Manchester Madonna* (see Fig. 58), he can be distinguished by his peculiar garment.

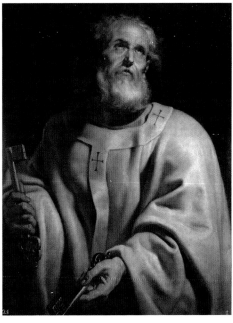

Fig. 110: Peter Paul Rubens, *Saint Peter*, 1610–12. St. Peter is shown here as pope with his attributes, the keys to heaven.

(The two figures in the painting also differ by the appearance of their foreheads—enlarged in the case of the young John the Baptist. This is not at all an identifying trait of the saint, but the child who posed for the painting may have had the frontal bossing of thalassemia, a disease endemic around the Mediterranean Sea.)

Some attributes refer to the person's deeds (Fig. 111): St. Daniel is usually seen with a lion, representative of those he tamed; St. Nicholas carries three purses or gold balls, symbolizing the gifts he bestowed on the poor (and the dowries of three daughters in a particular story); St. Francis of Assisi, who lived among the animals, is usually depicted with a bird. In other cases, the attribute is a direct allusion to the saint's name. St. Agnes, for example, is usually shown with a lamb (*agnus* in

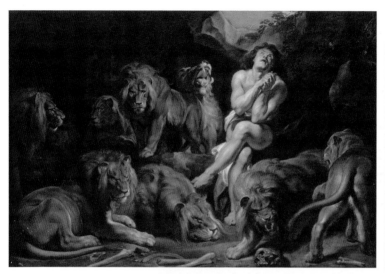
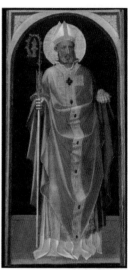
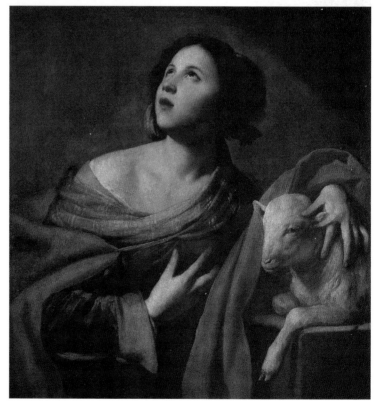

Fig. 111: Saints and their attributes. *From left to right:* Peter Paul Rubens, *St. Daniel in the Lion's Den* (detail), circa 1614; Gherardo di Jacopo Starnina, *Saint Nicholas of Bari,* circa 1422; Massimo Stanzione, *Saint Agnes,* 1635.

Latin). More commonly, the attribute refers to their martyrdom, and in a sometimes strange twist, the cause they represent: St. Agatha, the patron saint of breast cancer and mastectomy, carries her two breasts on a plate. St. Lucia, the patron saint of the blind, carries her two eyes.

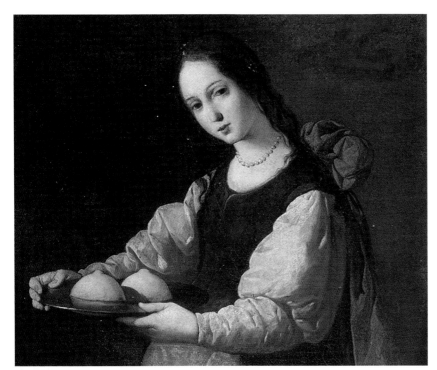

Fig. 112: Martyr saints and their attributes, both a depiction of how they died, and who they protect. *Right:* Francisco de Zurbarán, *Saint Agatha,* circa 1630; *bottom left:* Domenico di Pace Beccafumi, *Santa Lucia* (St. Lucia), 1521; *bottom right:* Student of Lucas Cranach the Elder, *Heiligen Erasmus* (St. Erasmus), circa 1510.

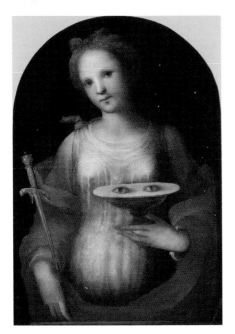

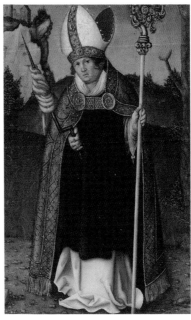

St. Elmo (or Erasmus) is usually shown with his intestines coiled on a windlass, a reminder of how he was tortured, and what he represents: he is the patron saint of abdominal pain and colic (Fig. 112). St. Apollonia, whose teeth were pulled or shattered to make her renounce her faith, is represented with a tooth or tongs. She is the patron saint of dentists and toothaches.

Although many of the origin stories of these saints have long been lost, the concept of attributes and symbolism is part of our common heritage. Illiteracy may have been eradicated in most developed countries, but reading grade levels vary widely, and medical terminology can be intimidating even to the well educated. Moreover, our world is increasingly global and multicultural, and language barriers are problems encountered daily by patients and healthcare professionals.[1] Nonverbal communication is not always easy in medicine, but when it works, it can tear down walls. And just as finding common reference points improves communication, the best medical and scientific illustrations take full advantage of visual cues that are universal, unequivocal, and easy to understand.

Christoph Niemann, a renowned illustrator and graphic designer who has been widely published in the *New Yorker,* the *New York Times Magazine,* and many other outlets, perfectly describes the relationship between reader and illustrator in his 2018 TED talk.[2] While it is the illustrator's task to find the correct way to communicate a concept as efficiently as possible, the success of an illustration depends greatly on the language most of us don't even realize we understand: the visual language. This visual language, he argues, is atavistic and innate, or at least intuitive: we associate certain images with more complex concepts than these images represent, so that the artist can use shortcuts, allowing the audience to fill in the gaps. Of course, it assumes that the entire audience has had the same experiences, and can draw from the same collective memory. This is not unlike the attributes of saints, when people could either remember stories about each martyr, or would associate an attribute with a name. The Eastern Orthodox Church, in particular, is known for the stylistic representation of saints and their attributes in the form of icons. The term *icon* (from the Greek εἰκών, or *eikon, image*) has had many meanings in history, but the modern icon, or symbol, has a lot in common with the religious icon: both are quick-and-easy ways to identify a person or concept through stylistic symbolism that we all understand.

Some concepts are so universal that they transcend not only cultures but centuries, even as the original object that is represented has long disappeared. Measuring time by watching sand slowly trickle

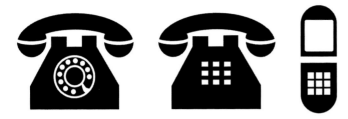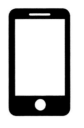

Fig. 113: Pictogram of a phone. *From left to right:* the old rotary phone is updated to a touch-tone one, but the horn still looks antiquated, as modern phones have evolved from flip phones to smartphones.

down is a thing of the distant past, but the hourglass itself remains a near-universal symbol of time or waiting. The pictogram for alarm or sound is a church bell, even though there is very little analog ringing anymore. Other icons or symbols have changed over time as our perception of its image has changed. Technology is moving at a dizzying speed, and modernizing an icon may seem futile. It can sometimes even be more befuddling than the original, antique symbol. In some computer operating systems and applications, the hourglass was replaced by a wristwatch, sometimes with moving hands. Of course, almost no one wears a wristwatch anymore, and if they do, it is more likely to be a digital than an analog one. The icon for the *Save* command in some programs is a diskette—never mind that that icon was introduced long after diskettes had become obsolete. The symbol for a rotary telephone may have been updated to a touch-tone one (Fig. 113), but the handset remains antiquated.

The Symbols of Medicine

Centuries ago, doctors were mostly contemplative diagnosticians, with very limited tests at their disposal. As mentioned in chapter 2, examining the color, the odor, and even the taste of body fluids—urine in particular—played a central role as microscopy and electrolyte analysis were not yet available. Treatment was limited to salves and other plant-based medicine, much of it of unproven benefit. In Christian iconography, the twin martyrs St. Cosmas and St. Damian, both physicians who offered free services to the poor, are represented with their attributes: an urn or medicine box, and a flask, symbolizing the diagnostic value of examining urine (Fig. 114). Centuries later, this proto-urinalysis would feature prominently in paintings of doctors by Gerrit Dou, Frans van Mieris, and many other Dutch artists (Fig. 115). As their methods improved, doctors produced ever more sophisticated diagnoses. The various sounds emitted by the heart and lungs gave clues to underlying conditions like pneumonia, pleuritis, atrial fibrillation,

Below, left: Fig. 114: *Saint Côme et Saint Damien* (St. Cosmas and St. Damian), in *Grandes Heures d'Anne de Bretagne* (Book of hours of Anne of Brittany). St. Cosmas holds a flask of urine, symbol of the diagnostician, and St. Damian has an urn of salves, representing medicinal herbs and plants.

Right, and below, right: Fig. 115: Gerrit Dou, *Doctor,* 1653. Seventeenth-century physicians had few diagnostic tools at their disposal. Looking at a patient's urine was one of them. The doctor would examine it for color and turbidity, as well as smell and taste. (Note the book in the foreground—Vesalius's *De Humani Corporis Fabrica,* volume 1, open on p. 163.)

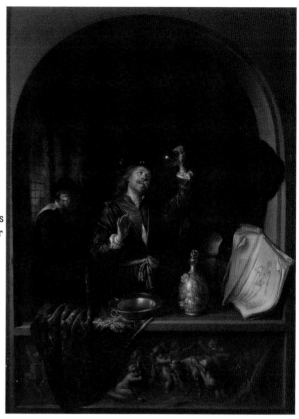

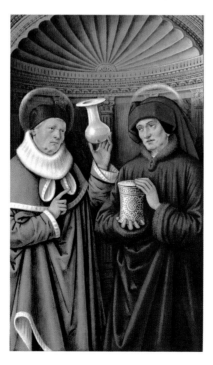

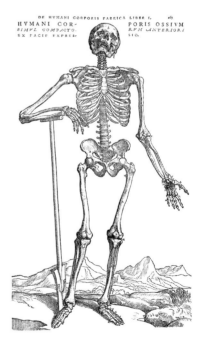

valvular disease, pericarditis, and heart failure. The introduction of the stethoscope by Laennec in 1816 represented a significant step forward. While his invention (essentially, a rolled-up sheet of paper) bears little resemblance to modern stethoscopes, it symbolized a new era in clinical medicine, and is today a universal icon representing physicians (Fig. 116). It is not the only shortcut to illustrate a doctor, however: like many other popular representations, we owe some of our modern medical iconography to 1950s comics. Thus, a cartoon doctor is often shown wearing a head mirror—an instrument that is foreign to most medical students today, and even in its heyday was limited mostly to ophthalmologists and otolaryngologists (ENT doctors). Why this device came to represent all doctors is unclear,[3] but there is at least one iconic painting that may have served as an example—Otto Dix's 1926 portrait of Dr. Mayer-Hermann (Fig. 117).

The archetype for doctor is a figure wearing a stethoscope or a head mirror; the symbol for hospital or ambulance is often a building or a vehicle with a red cross, at least in the Western (Christian) world. Although it is a ubiquitous shortcut for anything medical, its

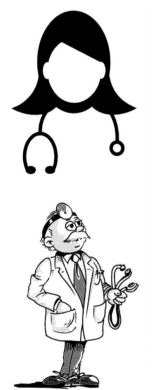

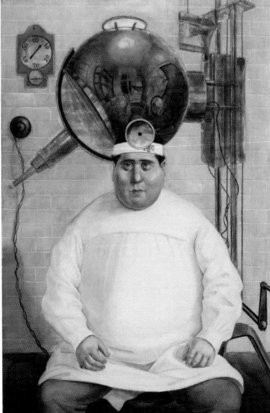

Left: Fig. 116: Pictogram and cartoon character of doctors, represented by their attributes: the stethoscope (*top*) and the head mirror.

Right: Fig. 117: Otto Dix, *Dr. Mayer-Hermann,* 1926. Possibly a source for the head mirror as a symbol of doctors in popular culture and comic books, even though the head mirror is rarely used today. (Copyright ARS, NY and The Museum of Modern Art/ Licensed by SCALA/ Art Resource, NY.)

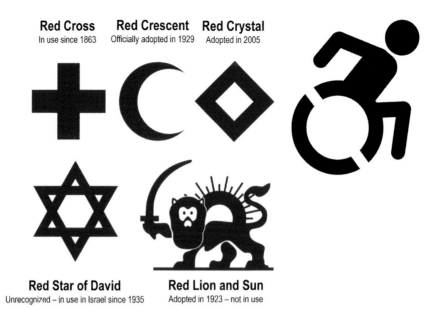

Red Cross
In use since 1863

Red Crescent
Officially adopted in 1929

Red Crystal
Adopted in 2005

Red Star of David
Unrecognized – in use in Israel since 1935

Red Lion and Sun
Adopted in 1923 – not in use

origin is unknown to many: it is the opposite of the Swiss flag (white cross on red background), which reflects, alternatively, the uniform and neutral symbol of aid as established at the 1864 Geneva (Switzerland) Convention, a design proposed by Louis Appia and Guillaume Henri Dufour, two Swiss founding members of the International Red Cross Committee, or to honor Henry Dunant, Swiss humanitarian and spiritual father of the Red Cross. Although the red cross has no direct ties with Christianity, the white cross of the Swiss flag does. This stirred controversy because of its Eurocentric, Christian slant. Turkey was the first Muslim country to object to the global use of the cross. Other countries followed suit. Therefore, the emblem of this worldwide organization may be a red crescent (the official name of the organization is the International Red Cross and Red Crescent Movement), a red Star of David, a red lion and sun, or a red crystal (Fig. 118). Other examples of insensitive iconography include the depiction of a doctor as a man or a nurse as a woman, or the implication that people with disabilities are helpless. The classic icon for handicap access is a person in a wheelchair. While this is a quick way to point to a ramp or accessible parking spot, it can be used inappropriately as well. Using the icon on a help button is particularly egregious, for example: it suggests that needing help is a handicap, or that a handicapped person automatically needs assistance. Fig. 119's version of the symbol shows a person self-propelling his or her own wheelchair: clearly, the person is doing just fine without anybody's help. Thus, universally recognized icons and symbols have a cultural value, too, and are yet another example of how medical and scientific illustration, like other forms of visualization, have a social responsibility.

Icons and pictograms (not only those used in medical illustration and scientific visualization) can be obsolete, inappropriate, or insensitive, like the Red Cross emblem or the image of a male doctor. They can also be confusing or unclear. This is especially true now that icons as shortcuts are more popular than ever. Our society has become overburdened with data and information. Simple images allow us to quickly determine what we view as important, so that we can select how best to utilize our precious time. Icons are also more useful than ever because of limited space. Not only are our lives becoming more connected, but our viewing space and digital real estate is shrinking. From desktop and laptop computers, we have mostly shifted to tablets, phones, and watches, and the print has become increasingly small. Stylizing or simplifying the icon is therefore important. However, there is danger in oversimplification, and creating clear, unequivocal icons is an art. Christoph Niemann facetiously created an "abstract-o-meter" to illustrate this point.[4] On a sliding scale from most realistic to most abstract, he illustrates the best way to convey love in a single icon. Make the illustration too realistic, and a beating heart violently pierced by a sharp projectile does not really evoke romance. Reducing it to its simplest geometric forms—a red square crossed by a black horizontal line—makes it utterly incomprehensible. Somewhere in the middle of these two extremes is the ubiquitous heart-shaped form with stylized arrow that represents all things love. The ideal icon—the sweet spot between too realistic and too abstract—can vary greatly. It depends on the clarity of the subject. Brightness, for example, can be represented by the sun, which can be depicted with any lack of detail—down to a simple open circle—without losing its meaning.

Creating shortcuts to simplify a more complex concept depends on the intended audience as well. It draws from our collective consciousness, including our cultural baggage. Fig. 120 shows several seemingly random expressions, ranging from a wry smile to a stern gaze. If given the information that these represent classic paintings, viewers might recognize these as the iconic expressions they are associated with: Mona Lisa's enigmatic smile, Edvard Munch's *The Scream,* and Grant Wood's *American Gothic,* an austere father-and-daughter portrait (Fig.

Fig. 120: Various expressions, from a wry smile to a stern look. They may seem random, but they can also be a reference to famous portraits in classical art.

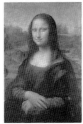

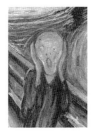

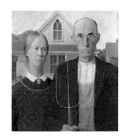

Fig. 121: When told that the faces in Fig. 120 represent classic paintings, viewers may recognize Leonardo da Vinci's *Mona Lisa* (*left*), Edvard Munch's *The Scream* (*middle*), and Grant Wood's *American Gothic* (*right*).

Over here,
I found bacon!

Juggler giving up
on his dream

Left: Fig. 122: Confusing or ambiguous signs are often seen in the arcane world of washing instructions. *Top:* The symbol for letter, envelope, or mail (*left*) looks a lot like the washing instruction to *hang clothing to dry* (*right*); *bottom:* The symbol to alert to the danger of acid or caustic injury (*left*) resembles the instruction to *hand wash only* (*right*).

Right: Fig. 123: Fun with pictograms. The jokes work because everyone is familiar with the symbols for swimming pool and trash bin.

121). Da Vinci's and Munch's masterpieces are almost universally recognizable. While *American Gothic* is a national treasure, however, that painting may be less well known on the other side of the Atlantic. The *Aha!* moment one has when instantly recognizing the context around an icon can easily become a *Huh?* reaction for the wrong audience. In an effort to simplify, symbols can also take on ambiguous meanings. Take the Byzantine world of laundry symbols and washing instructions, for example. The icon for *Hang clothing to dry* is almost identical to the universal symbol for a letter, email, or mail. The warning sign for acid or caustic substance looks a lot like the instruction for *Hand wash only* (Fig. 122). Obviously, this confusion can lead to dangerous situations. And of course, ambiguity can also spark comedy, like the symbols for swimming pool (*Over here, I found bacon!*) and trash bin (*Juggler giving up on his dreams*) (Fig. 123).

How Do You Draw Diabetes?

With all this in mind, how best to represent medical conditions and treatments? Organ-specific diseases are usually relatively straightforward, although the icon will depend on the audience's knowledge of anatomy. Orthopedics, cardiology, and neurology are easy to illustrate—everyone can recognize bones, the heart, or the brain. Kidney and lungs are easily recognizable as well, even in their more stylized versions (Fig. 124). Other conditions may be more difficult to represent, even if they are well known and common. Diabetes is a disease of the pancreas, whereby islet cells do not produce or release enough insulin to regulate blood sugar levels. To diabetologists, depicting the pancreas may make perfect sense. However, most laypeople do not know what the pancreas looks like and may not associate diabetes with the pancreas. What, then, does the concept of diabetes evoke? Diabetic patients can't eat too much sugar, since they cannot metabolize it correctly, placing them at risk for hyperglycemia. Depicting a spoonful of sugar or a pastry could hint at diabetes, but these images are obviously not specific to the disease and can be ambiguous. Type 2 diabetes is associated with obesity, but showing an overweight person can be as ambiguous as it is offensive. Diabetes can lead to kidney failure and vascular problems, including leg ulcers and arterial blockages, which can eventually lead to gangrene, amputation, or the need for arterial bypass. It can affect the peripheral nerves as well, sometimes causing pressure ulcers because patients can't feel parts of their body. It can lead to vision problems and even to stroke and heart disease. Most of these effects of diabetes are not specific to the disease itself, and many symptoms are difficult or gruesome to illustrate. A common depiction of diabetes relies on the diagnostic test, and on the now common sight

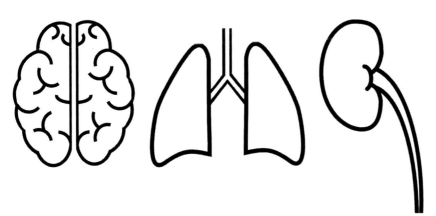

Fig. 124: Stylized icons of organs as stand-ins for their respective specialty. *From left to right:* brain (neurology), lungs (pulmonology), kidney (nephrology).

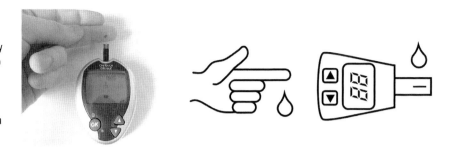

of personal glucose meters, whereby a patient analyzes a drop of blood using a small electronic device. Most people recognize the glucometer itself, or understand that a fingerstick blood sample is used (Fig. 125). As with the cartoon faces in Fig. 121, understanding a shortcut depends heavily on what the viewers already know—they must be good at filling the gaps. Good illustrators must therefore predict what is common knowledge and what isn't, and know their audience. They must also be aware of context. The icon of a light bulb on a control panel indicates light or brightness; in a different context, it can signify an idea or an inspiration—a figurative light is suddenly turned on, making it clear to see. The heart symbol can signify love and, by extension, like, for example, a preferred treatment. It can represent the general specialty of cardiology, or a more specific aspect of cardiovascular physiology such as the heartbeat or, by questionable extension, blood pressure. On a restaurant menu, it can indicate lean cuisine, which is good for your heart. Likewise, the icon of a human brain can be a shortcut for thought in a heading for puzzles or brain teasers; it can refer to the field of neurology, psychiatry, or neurosurgery; in traumatology, it points to head injuries, while it refers to brain tumors in oncology or brain development in fetal medicine. Of course, these concepts are not limited to the visual arts: whether we call it pars pro toto, metonymy, or synecdoche, our language is full of examples where we use a body part to mean an entire person (head count), a place (like the Vatican) as a stand-in for its occupant, or materials, such as brass and strings, to describe entire orchestra sections.

The Ninth Art Form

It is pretty obvious that medical illustration has its roots in classic art. The early medical illustrators were artists and painters first. Van Calcar and other draftsmen's anatomic plates for Vesalius's *De Humani Corporis Fabrica,* de Lairesse's for Professor Bidloo, and van Rymsdyk's for the Hunter brothers are all masterpieces that are as beautiful to look at as they are scientifically accurate. As medical knowledge evolved, however, science became less contemplative (anatomy) and more procedural. Advances in physiology, pharmacology, embryology, and biochemistry paved the way for evidence-based treatments. With the advent of anesthesia, aseptic techniques, and a refined understanding of human pathophysiology, increasingly daring and complex surgical interventions could be performed. This moved the realm of medicine and medical illustration from static and observational to dynamic and interventional. Where classic art had been a perfect learning ground for the field of medical illustration, the modern era of medicine required an additional source of inspiration for illustrators.

Enter the ninth art. The term originated in the 1960s in France, where it is still used to describe the world of comics and graphic novels (the six classical arts, according to Hegel's *Aesthetics,* were architecture, sculpture, painting, literature, music, and dance; cinema became known as the seventh art form, and television and media in general are the eighth). Comics (*manga* in Japan, or BD, short for *bandes dessinées,* in the French-speaking world) combine literary narratives with visual arts, but they introduce a new element: dynamic annotations. The light bulb, to denote inspiration, originated in the comics, and is universally understood as a sudden event that turns fumbling in obscurity into instant clarity. It not only illustrates the bright idea, but the immediacy of the feeling as well. What separates comics from static art is the conveyance of motion, action, and dynamism. A fast-moving car on a dirt road leaves behind a cloud of dust. By extension, fast-running comics characters are depicted with a small cloud behind them, usually accompanied with a swoosh or motion lines (annotations that also find their roots in animated cartoons, themselves inspired by early cinema). To show directional motion, the comic book artist may even add repeated partial outlines of where the character just was in an attempt to show an entire moving sequence in one image. Emotions can be expressed with radial lines, sweat droplets, smoke, or thunderclouds—all shortcuts to evoke an action or a mood in one illustration. While medical illustrations don't typically depict anger or anxiety, they may need to suggest motion, dynamism, a logical progression, or an acute event. Good medical illustrations also collapse time, showing successive actions or events in a single image (Fig. 126). To enhance the value of such an image, the use of comics-inspired annotations is frequent, and, thanks to our collective cultural baggage, we understand these archetypal symbols (see Fig. 8 in the introduction).

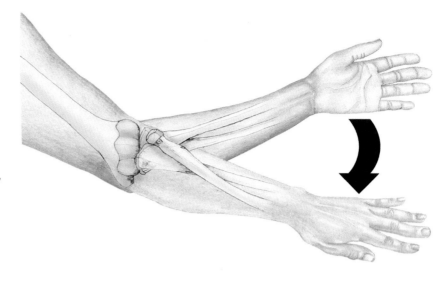

Fig. 126: Kuukua A. Wilson, The mechanics of wrist motion. As the hand goes from supination to pronation, the radius crosses the ulna. Using a technique borrowed from cinema and comics, the illustrator superimposes two positions of the forearm, creating the illusion of motion.

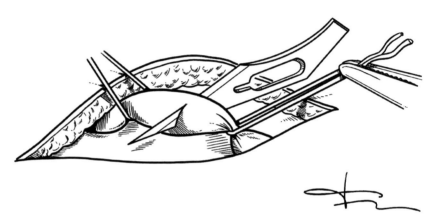

Fig. 127: Simplifying illustration to improve readability (technique of venotomy, or how to incise a vein). The iconic shape of a no. 11 scalpel blade is sufficiently recognizable without the need to add a knife handle, which would obscure or clutter the illustration; any surgeon knows not to use the blade alone, but to hold it by its handle.

Since medical illustration is, in essence, a form of visual communication, the goal is to be effective and not necessarily artistic. Intricate, detailed, full-color lifelike illustrations can be impressive, and depending on the context and the audience, extremely helpful. However, simplification is often a goal in itself. A good medical illustration can be more helpful than a vivid photograph because it purposefully highlights important aspects while muting extraneous information.[5] Similarly, a simplified pen-and-ink drawing can be more effective than a grayscale painting of the subject (compare Fig. 39 and Fig. 89, for example). Omitting certain aspects of the scene can add even more clarity: depicting a very recognizable surgical blade is as effective as showing the entire scalpel, handle and all, and critical structures are not obscured by unnecessary clutter (Fig. 127). Using a clear symbol may be more effective than drawing a true-to-life object or organ.

This is even truer when the exact shape of the structures to be depicted is not actually known. In cellular biology, for example, cells and cell organelles are often depicted schematically, with just enough visual cues to help the reader: the cell membrane of dendritic cells has spiky projections (see Fig. 104); mitochondria are elongated organelles with a double membrane and radiator-like pattern; and ribosomes resemble early video-game characters, chain-assembling amino acids into linear strings of proteins—never mind that some of these images, based on light-microscopic examination, turn out to be shaped very differently when examined in three dimensions using scanning electron microscopy. The correct shapes of many of these microscopic and molecular structures have since been elucidated—sometimes with the help of medical illustrators, as detailed in chapter 4—but the simplistic depiction remains a useful shortcut when explaining a process, a disease, or a biochemical reaction.

SciViz

For centuries, medical illustration was synonymous with the macroscopic representation of the human body and its organs. With the rapid expansion of biologic knowledge, this description has become too limited, and a more common term is *scientific visualization.* For many reasons, including the need to simplify complex concepts and "big data" and the arbitrary depiction of unknown structures, scientific visualization (SciViz, for the initiated) relies equally on lifelike images, icons, and symbols. A recent phenomenon has seen the merger of all the elements of the visual language into an instantly recognizable and usable tool: the visual abstract. The visual abstract was officially introduced around 2016 but is only the newest iteration of infographics, this time geared toward social media, and as an answer to the unmanageable amount of scientific data that clinicians and scientists must deal with. It is also an evolutionary way to summarize scientific articles.[6] Most medical and scientific articles contain an abstract, a structured summary of the study described in the paper. These abstracts, which scientific journals typically restrict to about 250 to 300 words, are a useful way to scan an article: Is it relevant to me? Does the methodology appear sound? Are the conclusions surprising, controversial, or already well known? We usually read a scientific paper's abstract first to get the gist, rather than reading the article from its introduction to its conclusion, and although they would probably deny it, most physicians don't even read the whole abstract at first but jump directly to its final summarizing paragraph or to the figures. (Not that this behavior is limited to scientific literature. David Remnick, the editor of the *New Yorker,* has quipped that 95 percent of readers go to the cartoons first, and the other 5 percent are lying.[7]) In an age of 280-character tweets and a constant competition for attention and clicks, it was only a matter of time before the short abstract was made even shorter and less text-heavy.

The visual abstract, in its current form, is used by a fast-growing number of scientific journals and medical societies to disseminate knowledge to their readers or members, usually (but not always) via social media.[8] Purists may see these "cartoons" as one more proof of the dumbing down of our society, but the visual abstract serves many purposes. Users of social media know that a post that contains an image is much more likely to be noticed and opened than a text-only one. Scientific journals want to increase their visibility and readership, and click rate is obviously important to them. If the visual abstract is simple to understand, catchy in its graphic design, and informative enough, it will lead the reader to the abstract or the full article—a win for the journal. The reader gets something out of it as well: the number of scientific journals available to the clinician has ballooned in recent years, and the arrival of predatory and bogus publications that lack adequate peer review has only made it worse. How, then, is a clinician to find the important and useful science amid the clutter? Recognizing the provenance of a post from a reputable journal can be very helpful. A quick scan of the image can help the readers decide whether the paper it represents may be of interest to them, or can help them skip it altogether if the topic or information is irrelevant. It does not replace the abstract or the full article, but it helps readers scan the rapidly changing landscape of medicine more efficiently—and what is wrong with that?

The perfect visual abstract does not (yet) exist. Andrew Ibrahim, MD, is credited as the originator of the visual abstract in its most re-cent form, and as the author of the first primer on the subject.[9] Much like the crowdsourcing wiki approach in many other fields, the visual abstract canon is a living document that is constantly evolving. To be effective, it needs to adhere to certain principles. These principles are self-evident, but the way to achieve them may be a matter of personal preference and likely to change over time. Text should be reduced to a minimum. Whereas the full paper it refers to may contain hard, detailed data, the visual abstract displays the essence of the study, the general idea. Sometimes text or numbers are the best way to convey that message, but often an image will be more effective in expressing

Data-driven comparison of operating room headgear

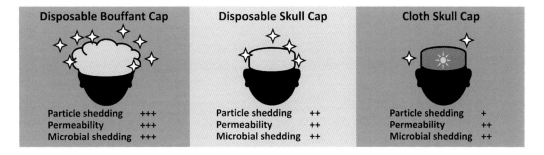

Markel TA, et al. Hats Off: A Study of Different Operating Room Headgear Assessed by Environmental Quality Indicators. J Am Coll Surg 2017;225:573-81.

a trend, a difference in outcome between groups, or a striking result. The most effective image communicates a concept and does not just function as filler. In the surgical headgear example (Fig. 128), a study looked at the relative risk of contamination between various head coverings worn in an operating room. This may sound like a strange and esoteric study, but it was generated following a controversy involving the Association of Operating Room Nurses (AORN) and the American College of Surgeons, two of the leading professional organizations representing healthcare providers in the United States.[10] Several years ago, AORN issued a set of guidelines recommending that all operating room personnel wear a bouffant cap to make sure that all hair was tucked away. They argued that the skullcap type of headgear, more commonly favored by (male) surgeons, left a portion of hair exposed, and therefore posed a greater risk of contamination in the operating room. The American College of Surgeons disagreed, citing lack of scientific evidence. This seemingly innocuous statement caused quite a stir and highlighted something of a power play between the two professional bodies. The fact that bouffant caps are more often worn by women and skullcaps by men added a gender issue to the nurse-doctor rivalry. Troy Markel and colleagues studied the concentration of particles and bacterial material on the outside of the various headgear, and showed that the bouffant caps, which are flimsier and therefore more porous, in fact shed more particles than the other types.[11] The visual abstract in Fig. 128 illustrates these results with simple silhouettes and distinctive features of each type of headgear, and the number of stars floating around each gives a visual representation of the differences in shedding. The text goes into more detail about what was specifically studied; the three icons give a quick indication of which surgical hat is best. Paradoxically, the cloth skullcap, which many hospitals had

Fig. 128: Visual abstract: A simple set of three pictograms with minimal text to summarize a scientific study. Here, the controversy about which operating room head gear (bouffant cap, disposable or cloth skull cap) is the cleanest.

banned because of the AORN guidelines, performed best. A curious surgeon gets the crux of the study at a glance, and can then decide to read the specifics of the study. And the other 99.9 percent of doctors can move on and ignore this niche research, spending their precious time on more important science.

Not only should the images and the text be complementary, the whole visual abstract must be clear, concise, and uncluttered. This is important because of the typical viewing platform. Portable devices have a small screen, and an icon must be recognizable even when severely shrunken. If the image is too detailed, its nuances will be lost when reduced in size—or worse, the icon may look like something completely different (Fig. 129). Similarly, the sparse words or numbers must be legible on a smartphone's screen, which significantly limits the amount of text in a visual abstract. Layout itself can help convey a message, as in this visual abstract offering the various forms of doctor-child-parent relationships (Fig. 130). The article asked where a pediatrician should stand when there is an intergenerational conflict. Should they side with the parents? After all, you wouldn't want to undermine parental authority. Or should they choose the side of the child, who deserves an advocate? The authors concluded that the wisest role for the pediatrician was to be a mediator by facilitating dialogue between child and parent in as objective a manner as possible. The visual abstract took advantage of the presence of three distinct scenarios for the same conundrum. As with the surgical cap abstract, repetition of a theme or a pictogram makes it easier to move from one panel to the other, as the reader expects the same structure every time. Representing two sulking figures (by suggesting folded arms and a forward-bent head) evokes conflict (the figure on the left is shorter *and* has a comparatively larger head, suggesting a child).

Fig. 129: When designing a pictogram, it is important to consider how it may be used and downsized to fit on a small display screen, like a smartphone or a watch. The symbol for *doctor* can be a stethoscope, but fine details may get lost when reduced in size. The stethoscope is no longer visible in the figure on the far right, possibly confusing the viewer.

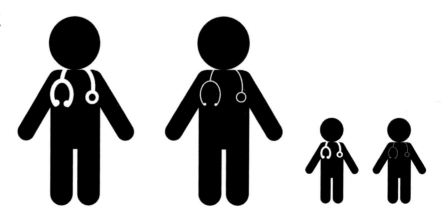

Pediatrician's Role when Child and Parents Disagree

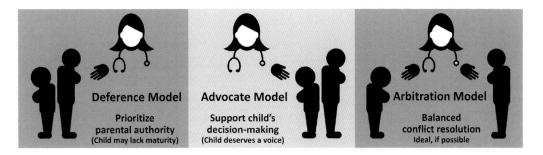

Deference Model
Prioritize parental authority
(Child may lack maturity)

Advocate Model
Support child's decision-making
(Child deserves a voice)

Arbitration Model
Balanced conflict resolution
Ideal, if possible

Sisk BA, et al. Navigating decisional discord: The pediatrician's role when child and parents disagree. Pediatrics 2017;139:e20170234.

They stand back-to-back in the first two panels, representing total disagreement: they literally don't see eye to eye. In the last panel, which recommends the ideal position for the pediatrician, they are still mad, but at least they are facing each other, suggesting a first step in conflict resolution. The action of the pediatrician is represented by her hand—alternately agreeing (open-hand gesture) with the parent and the child. In the last panel, the two open hands are less a symbol of agreement and more a suggestion of bridge building, inviting both to speak to each other.

Who is the visual abstract for? It clearly benefits the scientific journal or professional society that produces it: in social media posts, an image gets more clicks than plain text, and the visual abstract steers more readers to the journal's main site, which will hopefully translate into more subscribers. The use of iconic color schemes, logos, and other recognizable features enhances branding, and that alone may attract new readers: The *New England Journal of Medicine*'s red-and-white logo and distinctive font instantly evoke knowledge and wisdom. The reader may not be interested in a particular topic, but may trust the journal, which puts out only newsworthy and scientifically sound research. The visual abstract benefits readers, who may find it a useful tool to quickly weed through the clutter of research to identify those studies that truly matter to them. The visual abstract is also a very useful exercise for the person creating it, and may be a powerful form of teaching. In order to express a difficult scientific concept or medical diagnostic work-up, one must first understand it. If the goal is to separate the superfluous or peripheral from the essence, the visual abstract requires its creator to analyze the study first. It is the same exercise that is known in entrepreneurial circles as the elevator pitch. Attention span is short; can you summarize your project

Fig. 130: Visual abstract: Use of layout to tell a story. The only icons in the strip above are the child and parent (similar pictogram, but different height and head size), the doctor, and the doctor's hands. In the first two panels, the doctor's hand gesture indicates she agrees either with the parent (*left*) or the child (*middle*). The child and parent stand back-to-back, indicating conflict. In the third panel, the doctor stands between the two, but they are facing each other: they are now seeing eye-to-eye, and the doctor's hands show a conciliatory, inviting gesture.

effectively while you have potential investors' captive attention, and before they reach their floor and disappear forever? It is also akin to the medical illustrator's sketch, and why a medical illustration can be so much more effective than even the most detailed photograph: understand what needs to be shown, which details must be emphasized, which details are extraneous, and which viewing angle best depicts the crucial elements of the image. Although visual abstracts are primarily meant to direct viewer traffic, increase readership, and help consumers choose their reading material more efficiently, the act of creating a visual abstract can be a very useful learning tool. Because the artistic aspect of the pictograms is secondary, and as the internet offers a plethora of royalty-free icons and other images, it can be a very democratic method as well. Anyone can do it—no drawing skills necessary. Do you understand a research paper well enough to summarize its essence in three images?[12]

Of course, nobody says that a visual abstract must consist of only three panels, but that limitation turns out to be ideal for several reasons. Most research studies, grant proposals, and journal articles are structured in a similar fashion. After an introduction that highlights the background of the research, authors detail (1) the methods of the research, (2) the results of the study, and (3) the interpretation of data, typically headlined as *Discussion* or *Conclusions*. Structuring a visual abstract in the same way will be familiar to most scientific readers as

Fig. 131: The rule of three in comedy: setup, response (or pause), punch line. This principle is engrained in our communal psyche and makes a visual abstract (with its three repetitive panels) intuitive to read.

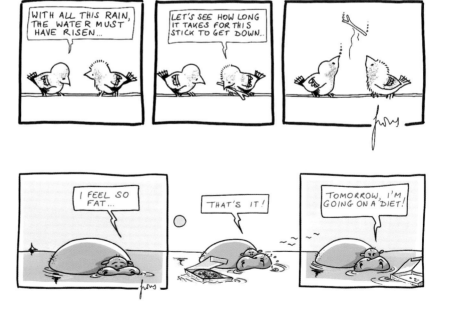

they view the panels sequentially. This natural progression reduces the need to explain how the visual abstract should be read, and the viewer knows intuitively that the last panel (the one on the right in Western languages) shows the conclusions. Three is also the maximum number of images for a visual abstract to be readable at reduced size. Since they exist mainly through social media, the small-screen format limits the amount of horizontal information display. Given the constraints of a 16:9 ratio (wide-screen) format, each of the three panels is roughly a square; increase the number of panels, and they become narrower, making it difficult to display more than a number or a few letters of text. Finally, there may be something more atavistic about a three-panel visual abstract. This "trinity" is also the basis of many comic strips (Fig. 131) and a golden rule of comedy, from Monty Python to Looney Tunes.

Chapter 6

Grammar and Syntax of Medical Illustration

Visual language may be universally understood, but it has its own grammar and syntax. Even when they are unwritten, rules of visual communication allow the reader and the illustrator to be in sync. This, in turn, allows the illustrator to take shortcuts and expect the reader to fill in the gaps in the narrative. Creating the perfect medical illustration therefore requires the talent of the artist, as well as the visual intelligence of the reader: a true collaboration of two individuals through the intermediary of the image. Understanding how a medical or scientific illustration is created can help enlightened viewers in their reading of the image, and at the very least help them appreciate the science behind the art.

Just Like in the Movies

The first principle of a good (medical) illustration is that the viewer's point of view must be established and understood. The illustrator will have spent a lot of effort deciding on the angle and the approach to the subject that will give the most amount of useful information. Typically, the illustrator will have discussed all possible options with the collaborating surgeon, anatomist, or scientist. They know what needs to be highlighted, and the artist helps them achieve that goal.[1] If, as in the example of Fig. 132, the goal is to illustrate the extrahepatic biliary anatomy (the gallbladder, common bile duct, hepatic duct, and that portion of the left and right hepatic ducts that lies outside the

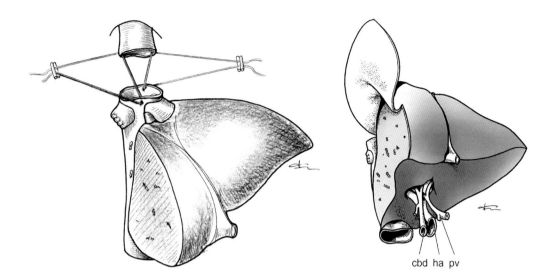

cbd ha pv

liver), the normal orientation of the liver as it lies in the abdominal cavity may not be the best angle. An upward view may be more logical, even if such a viewpoint is not realistic in real life (unless the liver is dissected out of the abdominal cavity). The goal is not to be as realistic as a photograph but to be accurate *and* didactic.

The degree of magnification and detail must be determined as well. Too much extraneous information only adds clutter that obfuscates the essence of the illustration. Too little detail or too great a close-up makes it difficult for the reader to understand the context, to know what is up and what is down. Illustrating a laparoscopic pyloromyotomy— the treatment for infants with the common condition known as pyloric stenosis—requires a magnified view of the organ. The important aspects of the procedure include the serrated instrument spreading the muscle fibers of the pylorus without damaging the underlying mucosa, which requires extreme close-ups of the pylorus (Fig. 133). Unfortunately, this close-up says nothing about where in the body the operation is taking place, or how the instrument is oriented in space. Adding a zoomed-out overview of the patient, the setup, and the orientation of the instruments can help situate the operation and make the instructional image more relevant (Fig. 134). If close-up and zooming out sound a lot like the movies, that is no coincidence. Whether in cinema, photography, illustration, or any other form of visual storytelling, orienting the viewers is crucial—they must know where they stand and have points of reference. This becomes even more important in a narrative: as the images and the scenes follow each other, the spectator must follow along. When there are transitions in the story (cutting from one movie scene to another, or from one character to the next),

Fig. 132: *Left:* Top-down view of partial liver transplantation, showing the anastomosis of the inferior vena cava and the hepatic veins (seen above the liver). *Right:* Same operation, viewed from below, which exposes the porta hepatis containing the bile ducts (cbd), the hepatic artery (ha), and the portal vein (pv).

Fig. 133: Laparoscopic pyloromyotomy in an infant. Close-up view shows the serrated instrument spreading the muscle fibers. The mucosa is visible underneath. Taken out of context, it is difficult to know what body part this represents.

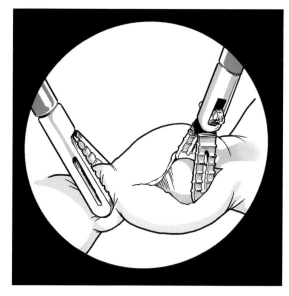

Fig. 134: Overview of the operative setup for a laparoscopic pyloromyotomy. It clearly shows the three instruments entering the distended abdominal cavity (*the telescope is in the middle*) and helps situate the close-up image in Fig. 133.

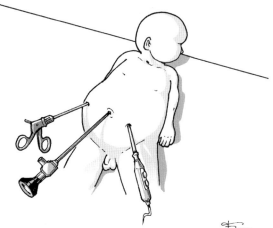

the spectator fills in these gaps. In graphic novels, medical illustrations, and many other forms of graphic narrative, these same rules apply. One of these, the 180-degree rule, dictates that from one scene to the next (or from one step to the next, when illustrating a surgical procedure), the point of view cannot change more than 180 degrees (Fig. 135). Let's say that an object or person stands to the left of another one (bottle and glass, respectively, in the example of Fig. 135); it is perfectly fine to cut to a close-up from the standpoint of the bottle, looking at the glass, and then from the glass's standpoint looking at the bottle, as long as the camera never rotates by more than 180 degrees along the axis between the two objects. Why? Because no matter whether the focus is on the bottle or the glass, the bottle always stands to the left of the glass. Transgress that imaginary line between the two objects and,

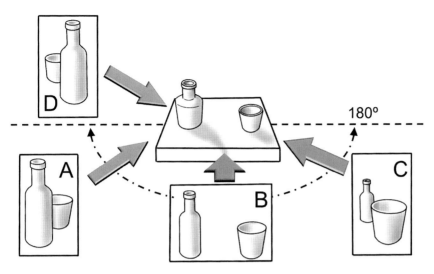

Fig. 135: The 180-degree rule. In cinematography, as in graphic narratives and even in laparoscopic surgery, first-person viewing requires that, when moving from scene to scene, the camera angle not change more than 180 degrees along the axis that connects two protagonists or landmarks. This will allow the viewer to understand the transitions: whether the emphasis is on the bottle or the glass, or both, the bottle is always to the left of the glass (A, B, and C). If the camera crosses the axis (D), the image is inverted: now the bottle is to the right of the glass.

suddenly, the positions seem inversed: The bottle magically appears to the right, not the left of the glass. In a series of scientific illustrations, the same rule may apply: for the reader to understand the progression of various steps (an operation, a biochemical pathway), they must intuitively grasp what successive images represent; the landmarks must be immediately identifiable, so that the reader can focus on the action itself without having to readjust to the surroundings. This 180-degree rule also happens to be very important in the performance (not just the depiction) of laparoscopic surgery—here, too, a single point of view (the camera and telescope) dictates what everyone sees, and that image must be logical. The camera represents the eye of the surgeon, and should therefore point in the general direction of the surgeon's field of vision. Place a surgeon on the *opposite* side of the camera (as when an assistant stands on the other side of the operating table) and everything becomes more difficult: the telescope captures a "paradoxical image," where left is right and right is left; when the camera pans in one direction, the image projected on the screen moves in the opposite direction for the surgeon's assistant, making efficient operative work almost impossible.

The more magnified and specialized the focus of an illustration, the more important it is to maintain a consistent viewing angle. As in the example of the pyloromyotomy, it is not uncommon to start a series of illustrations for an operation by showing the site of the surgical incision. An outline of an upright patient is a logical choice (Fig. 136A). However, the close-up details of the operations should be similarly oriented, especially if there are no recognizable landmarks (Fig. 136B). In the case of a thoracotomy to repair, for example, an esophageal atresia—when an infant is born with an interrupted esophagus—the normal intraoperative view is with the patient lying down, on the side

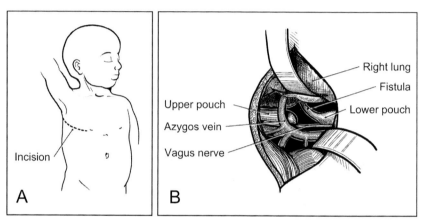

Fig. 136: Changing the angle of view between two steps of the same procedure is confusing for the viewer, particularly when extreme close-ups are used, or clear landmarks are missing. A: The outline of the incision for a thoracotomy to repair an esophageal atresia is clear on an upright view of the patient. The more logical field of view of a patient lying on an operating table, in B, shows the upper pouch (toward the patient's head) on the left and the lower pouch (toward the feet) on the right rather than top and bottom. The point of view has been rotated 90 degrees.

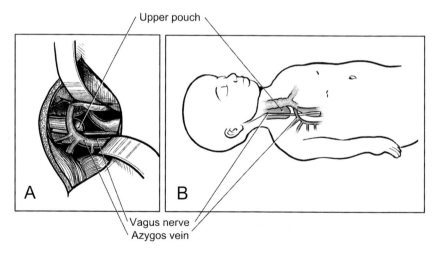

Fig. 137: In an illustration of the same operation as in Fig. 136, the close-up of the operating field (A) has the same orientation as the overall view of the patient (B).

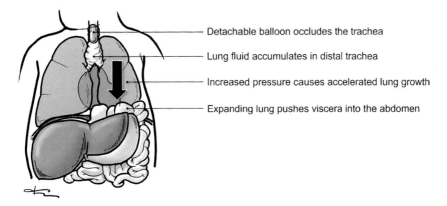

Detachable balloon occludes the trachea

Lung fluid accumulates in distal trachea

Increased pressure causes accelerated lung growth

Expanding lung pushes viscera into the abdomen

Fig. 138: Fetal tracheal occlusion to treat severe congenital diaphragmatic hernia in utero. This figure illustrates the complex concept of blocking the trachea of the fetus with a detachable balloon, causing lung fluid to build up and the expanding lungs to push the intestines and liver back into the abdomen through the hole in the diaphragm (arrow). The viewer naturally reads from top to bottom, which reflects the correct sequence of events.

(Fig. 136B). The intraoperative details make sense only if the viewer immediately understands where the head and the feet are, what is up and what is down (Fig. 137). As much as possible, each successive illustration should maintain the same hierarchy and orientation, or the changes in viewpoint should be clearly indicated.

Relying on conventions and instinct helps viewers to understand each separate image as well. In the Western world, we typically read from left to right and from top to bottom. Naturally, the viewer will be drawn to the top left area of a complex illustration, such as a biochemical cascade, an algorithm, a procedure with sequential steps, etc. A good illustrator will utilize these conventions to optimize the reading flow within the illustration. A telling example is the illustration of fetal tracheal occlusion, a seemingly "out there" treatment for severe diaphragmatic hernia before birth (Fig. 138). Congenital diaphragmatic hernia is a condition of the fetus and newborn whereby a portion of the diaphragm, the thin muscle that separates the thoracic cavity from the abdomen, fails to form. It occurs most commonly on the left side and, if severe, can be lethal: the abdominal contents (liver, intestines, stomach), which migrate into the chest cavity through the hole in the diaphragm, compress the fetus's lungs and prevents their full development. As a result, the newborn baby is unable to breathe normally and is at risk of dying. Operating directly after birth is possible, but the lungs are often so small that they cannot sustain life, even after the intestines have been returned to the abdomen and the diaphragmatic defect has been closed. Research into fetal surgery (operating on the fetus before birth by operating on the mother) has been conducted for several decades. In the 1990s, a significant breakthrough was made. It had been known that fetal lungs not only contain fluid (the fetus doesn't breathe through its lungs—oxygen comes through the placenta), but that they actively secrete this fluid into the future airspaces. What if, hypothetically, one blocked the trachea of the fetus? Would the fluid inside the lungs continue to accumulate and thereby cause the lungs to distend and grow? And if a diaphragmatic hernia was present and intestines and liver were herniated into the chest, would the growing lungs push these organs back into the abdomen? The short answer is that these assumptions proved to be correct.[2]

After years of fine-tuning the procedure, this type of intervention was offered to mothers who were pregnant with a fetus with diaphragmatic hernia.[3] A nifty technique was developed to block the trachea: a very small, detachable balloon, mounted on a carrier catheter, was introduced through the side port of a tiny endoscope passed into the fetus's airways and deployed in its trachea. The illustration of this complex concept in Fig. 138 utilizes the natural reading habits of the viewer. As we read the image from top to bottom, we first see the balloon in the trachea; the blockage causes the lung fluid to accumulate (which is suggested by the wide, distended trachea below the balloon), causing the lungs to grow and push abdominal content down (arrow), through the hole in the diaphragm, and back into the abdominal cavity. The top-to-bottom progression corresponds to the logical progression of the treatment as well.

Arrows

In the example above, the arrow indicates motion or movement—the intestinal loops that are being pushed down into the abdomen. Arrows are sometimes used to point at objects or structures, but purists feel that that should be avoided. Arrows are most effective when they indicate an action—movement, progression of time, structural shifts. Fig. 139 offers a perfect blend of passing time and physical motion. At ovulation, an egg cell is extruded from the ovary and captured by the fimbriae at the distal opening of the fallopian tube. As the top arrow indicates, the egg cell moves downstream through the oviduct and can be fertilized by sperm cells. Once fertilized, the egg cell starts to divide, first in two daughter cells, then four, then eight, all the while moving down the oviduct toward the uterus. Eventually, the morula (no more than a clump of cells) develops polarity (top-bottom differentiation)

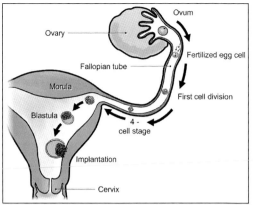

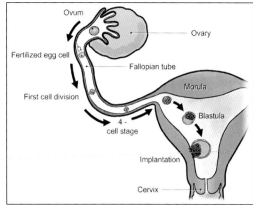

Left: Fig. 139: Early embryonal development from ovulation to implantation. The arrows show the temporal progression from unfertilized ovum through fertilization and early cell division to implantation in the uterus. The arrows also indicate a physical movement of the embryonic cell cluster from the fallopian tube into the uterus. *Right:* Fig. 140: Same sequence as in Fig. 139, this time showing the fallopian tube on the left. This allows the viewer to read the progression from left to right, which is more intuitive.

and its continuously dividing cells become more specialized, setting the stage for development into an early embryo. The arrows indicate the progression of time as the organism goes from single cell to embryo, as well as the physical progression from ovary to implantation into the wall of the uterus. The illustration is clear and explanatory, but the illustrator missed an opportunity to make the viewing even more intuitive: instead of showing the process from the right ovary to the uterus, it could have worked better from the left ovary: in that case (Fig. 140), the natural progression in time and space moves naturally, from left to right, as one would read a paragraph.

Of course, not all biochemical pathways or surgical interventions lend themselves to a top-to-bottom, left-to-right explanation. To help the reader along, other tricks may have to be used, such as numbering the steps (Fig. 141). In this example, an undescended testis is viewed from within the abdominal cavity, during laparoscopy. Visible are the bladder in the midline; the internal ring of the left inguinal canal to the left of the midline;

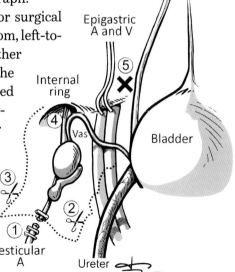

Fig. 141: Laparoscopic second-stage Fowler-Stephens orchidopexy. Not all concepts, reactions, processes, or operations can be illustrated by a logical top-to-bottom and left-to-right progression. Numbering the steps is an alternative solution for storytelling.

and numerous vascular and other structures one encounters during laparoscopic examination (the operative field is viewed through the telescope introduced at the level of the umbilicus, and we are looking down toward the pelvis; the lower portion of the anterior abdominal wall can be seen as it curves caudally toward the pelvis). Just as with the fetal treatment of congenital diaphragmatic hernia, the operation that is depicted here is a think-outside-the-box concept. Normally, the testes are located in the scrotum after birth (toward the end of gestation, the testis starts its journey from an intra-abdominal organ to an extra-abdominal one as it travels through the inguinal canal). The main blood supply to the testis comes from the renal artery, and the testicular artery is a very long vessel that accompanies the testis through its travels. If the testis doesn't descend properly, however, the testicular artery will not lengthen either. How, then, can the testis be brought down into the scrotum surgically if the artery that supplies its oxygen and nutrients won't reach? Leaving the testis in the abdomen is not a good idea—it won't function well, may twist and die, or may develop cancer. Faced with these choices, earlier generations of surgeons either removed the testis altogether, or tied off the testicular artery in the hope that the testis would survive anyway on collateral blood supply. Against all odds, this technique often resulted in testicular survival. The procedure was fine-tuned by tying off the artery first, allowing some ingrowth of other blood vessels to help the testis survive and bringing it down into the scrotum during a second operation, months later. The operation, which used to be performed through a large abdominal or flank incision, was adapted to a laparoscopic approach. The procedure, named after Dr. Robert Fowler and Dr. F. Douglas Stephens, is typically done in two laparoscopic stages: the first consists of placing a metal clip on the testicular artery.[4] The illustration in Fig. 141 describes the second-stage operation. The successive steps of this complex procedure are numbered to help the reader follow along. First, the previously clipped testicular artery is divided (1). Next, a swath of peritoneum covering the testis is incised; the hope is that new blood vessels will have formed on the surface of the peritoneum to help keep the testicle alive. This pedicle of peritoneum is developed by cutting down on it medially (2) and laterally (3), creating a peritoneal flap that is attached to the testis. To free up the testis at the distal end, the gubernaculum (4), a traction ligament that typically anchors the testis in the scrotum but is too long and lax here, is divided. Finally, the testis, freed from its tethers, can be brought into the scrotum by creating a window through the lower abdominal wall, at the point marked with an X (5).

The IKEA Model

The example in Fig. 141 shows an entire operation depicted in a single image. It gives the reader a rapid summary of what the procedure achieves, but may not be as effective as a step-by-step how-to manual. Illustrating a narrative continuum, such as a surgical procedure, can be difficult. Showing every single step amounts to a real-time movie of the operation—certainly accurate and complete, but long and tedious, particularly for complex procedures or concepts. As an example, Fig. 142 illustrates all the various steps of a laparoscopic appendectomy— from the identification of the appendix and the mesoappendix to the removal of the organ. It is certainly accurate, but it is lengthy and repetitive. The chronological steps of the operation read like a movie storyboard. However, there is no hierarchy between the various steps: they all seem to be equally important. Furthermore, the repetitiveness of the images sets the pace, like a metronome: all steps appear to take the same amount of time. While this storyboard could be useful (for example, as the basis for an animation of the procedure), it does not make optimal use of the reader's attention span. A better approach would be to highlight the important steps of the operation, caution the

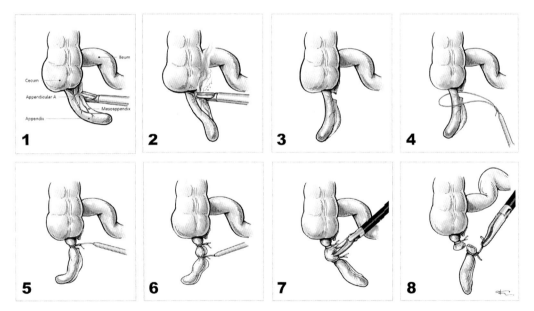

Fig. 142: Step-by-step laparoscopic appendectomy. The appendix and the mesoappendix are identified (1), an energy device (like the harmonic scalpel) is used to cauterize the mesoappendix (2), leaving the appendix devascularized (3). A first endoscopic ligature is passed around the base of the appendix (4) and cinched to occlude the appendix (5). A second ligature is placed 1 cm distal to the first one (6), and the appendix is divided between the two ligatures (7). It is then grasped and removed (8).

reader about critical aspects and priorities, and offer this in the least number of repetitions as possible. Of course, this idea is not limited to the surgical atlas, or even to scientific illustration: it is the goal of any how-to manual—to be exact, concise, and to the point.

Presenting clear, step-by-step illustrations that avoid redundancy, easily orient readers from figure to figure, alert them to critical parts in the assembly, and do this wordlessly is the hallmark of the IKEA instructions that accompany every one of their build-it-yourself products. This IKEA model is deceptively simple, but it is the well-thought-out result of all the principles mentioned above. Because paper and printing are expensive, it makes sense to reduce the number of illustrations to a bare minimum, avoiding any redundancy. Line drawings are better than photographs because the focus is not on the individual parts; rather, it is on the interaction between them, and the actions to connect them. Line drawings remove the distraction of the wood grain, the color or the texture of a particular component; the instructions emphasize small areas of these parts: a screw hole, a bolt, or a plug. These would more likely be overwhelmed by a large slab of fully rendered wood. Instead, the outline of the large pieces is there for context—to orient the customer to the correct positioning of the parts, the right hole for the right screw. Moreover, the instructions are wordless; at most, numbers indicate the sequence of images or the number of screws in the kit. For a company that is hugely successful worldwide, it was important not to require separate instructions in each language. The same instructional pamphlets can be used in Scandinavia, France, and the United States, saving time, effort, and money. So engrained is the IKEA model of instructional images that it has been spoofed many times, making it even more relatable in the global consciousness: the simple line drawings; the bold, no-nonsense sans-serif font; the quirky names with the occasional Ø, Ö, or Å (Fig. 143); and the ubiquitous (and always single) Allen wrench are instantly recognizable, and many have ridiculed and parodied it. Of course, the joke is on them because it only increases IKEA's brand visibility. An IKEA Australia April's Fools Day ad campaign even featured a supposed recall of "left-handed" Allen keys.[5]

The other iconic company that comes to mind when talking about easy-to-understand, wordless instruction sheets is LEGO, whose line drawings of building blocks in primary colors and step-by-step build-up figures of cars, trucks, houses, magical creatures, and entire sceneries are recognizable by people of all ages. It is probably not a coincidence that both companies are Scandinavian. Both would have realized early on that, in order to be a global company, you either had

GÅSTRØSTÖMY

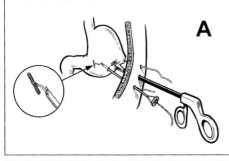
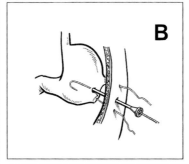
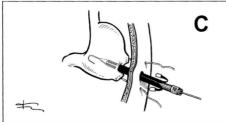
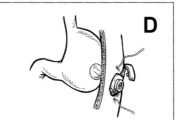

to switch to a world language (Danish or Swedish are clearly less universal than English), or find a way to be understood worldwide without words.

Time Compression

The genius of IKEA's instructional pamphlets is knowing the minimum number of images, and the minimum amount of detail for it to still make perfect sense. Reducing a continuous process, whether building a bookcase or performing an operation, to only its critical time points is the stuff of skilled illustrators. It also requires a perfect understanding of the process, and in the case of medical illustrators, a close collaboration with the physicians and scientists whose work is being described.[6] For the doctors themselves, collaborating with an illustrator requires them to express the crux of the process in simple terms and eliminate the extraneous, superfluous, or repetitious. An important tool in the illustrator's kit is compression of time. In the appendectomy example in Fig. 142, the steps illustrated in images 1 through 8 occur one after the other. It is possible to tell the exact same story without a movie-like series of images, relying on the visual language skills of the reader (Fig. 144). The first image draws attention to important landmarks like the mesoappendix and the appendicular artery, while the first step of the

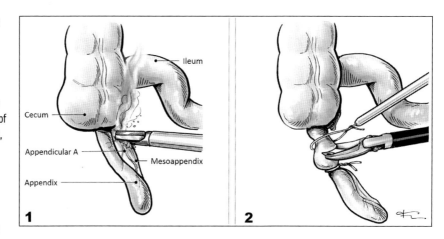

Fig. 144: Simplified illustration of a laparoscopic appendectomy, in only two images. Image 1 shows the devascularization of the mesoappendix, together with the anatomic landmarks; image 2 shows the first ligature already cinched down and the second ligature being placed while scissors divide the appendix. The reader should understand that these steps don't occur simultaneously but sequentially.

operation (cauterizing the mesoappendix) is taking place. The second image shows all successive steps simultaneously (division of the appendicular artery, placement of both endoscopic ligatures, and division of the appendix between the two ligatures) without the need to explain that this cannot all be done at the same time: even an inexperienced surgeon knows that opening the appendix has to occur *after* both ends have been tied off. Disruption of the time line and compression of multiple, successive steps into a single image requires more engagement on the part of the reader, who must fill in the gaps in the narrative and understand the correct sequence of events.

As with any didactic narrative, lesson, or conference, it is helpful to show what will happen, what is happening, and what has happened (Fig. 145). Choosing a time point in the middle of a procedure or step might simultaneously illustrate the anatomy *before* any intervention and the end result (Fig. 146).

That is the power of medical illustration: the ability to mold time and space to fit the narrative and to increase the didactic value of an image. The simultaneous visualization of several time points in a story requires compression of time and altering the time line hierarchy. A similar principle holds true when the scales of the subject vary widely. Several examples have already been cited where a close-up is preceded by a wide-angle view of the subject to better situate the action in context (see the thoracotomy in Figs. 136 and 137 and the pyloromyotomy in Figs. 133 and 134).

Another approach is to add close-up insets in the illustration to draw attention to certain details without losing sight of the overall subject: the inset in Fig. 143 shows a close-up of the anchor suture as it exits the needle. In some instances, it is even possible to illustrate

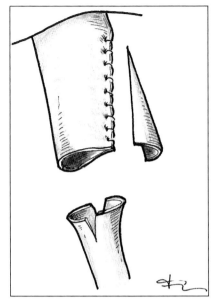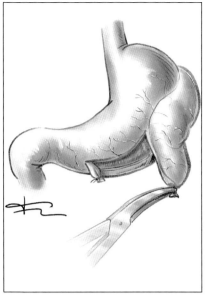

Left: Fig. 145: Pediatric liver transplantation. Discrepancy between adult-size vena cava of donor and smaller vena cava of recipient is addressed. Typically, the donor vein is trimmed to size by removing a wedge of the vein, while the recipient vein's end can be widened by making two incisions in "fish-mouth" fashion. A single illustration demonstrates the entire procedure, even though it requires sequential steps. Showing the discarded wedge of donor vein helps the reader understand the procedure.

Right: Fig. 146: A congenital duplication, consisting of an extra portion of intestinal tract. The duplication cyst has its own separate lumen but usually shares a muscularis layer with the native organ (here, the stomach). A single illustration shows the condition before resection (*right,* with visceral peritoneum covering stomach and cyst) and after removal (*left,* with cyst partially separated, revealing the joint muscle layer and peritoneum).

various aspects of the same subject, all at different scales, within the same image (Fig. 147). Using an extreme fish-eye lens effect, an illustration can achieve what no photograph can: a seamless transition from the macroscopic view of the heart, which pumps oxygenated blood through the aorta and its major blood vessels, through ever-smaller vascular branches, to the microscopic view of the individual cells that make up blood, and beyond to the ultrastructural view of individual molecules. Bending the rules of optics and perspective allows a single view to illustrate completely different dimensions all at once.

The essence of good medical illustration and scientific visualization in general is the use of a language that we all understand. It transcends nationalities and tongues; it is more understandable than arcane scientific jargon. Its goal is didactic efficiency, using image where many paragraphs would otherwise be needed, and a single illustration where an entire series of images would have been thought necessary. Time is compressed, repetition is avoided. In an age when high-definition photography is available and video documentation is ubiquitous (to say nothing of the computing power that can turn any diagnostic imaging test into a perfect three-dimensional picture), medical illustration provides an unparalleled ability to tell an entire story in the most effective manner possible. It does more than show a picture of reality (Fig. 148). It uses a combination of real images, augmented reality, annotations, conventions and symbols, and above all the creativity of an artist to reimagine the real world in order to better explain science (Fig. 149).

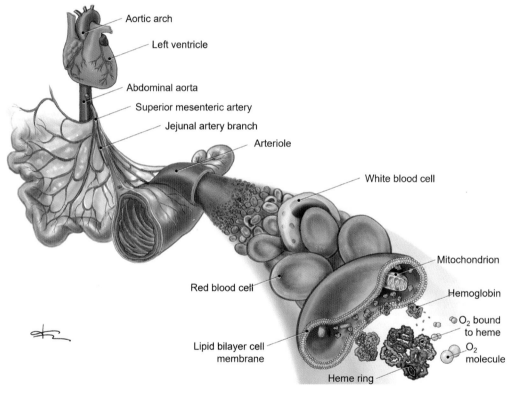

Aortic arch
Left ventricle
Abdominal aorta
Superior mesenteric artery
Jejunal artery branch
Arteriole
White blood cell
Mitochondrion
Hemoglobin
O_2 bound to heme
Red blood cell
O_2 molecule
Lipid bilayer cell membrane
Heme ring

Fig. 147: Oxygen transport by the blood: From the heart, through the aorta and its primary branches (like the superior mesenteric artery), blood travels through progressively smaller arterial branches to arterioles and capillaries that supply oxygen to the tissues. Oxygen is released from erythrocytes, specialized blood cells that do not contain a nucleus or organelles, except mitochondria, and are filled with hemoglobin (see Fig. 107). Each hemoglobin macromolecule consists of two α globin chains (in purple), and two β globin chains (in yellow); each globin chain contains a heme ring (in green). Oxygen binds to the heme rings of the hemoglobin molecule in the lungs, and is released in the peripheral tissues. As space and dimensions are compressed, the macroscopic view of large blood vessels and the cellular and molecular views can be combined in a single illustration.

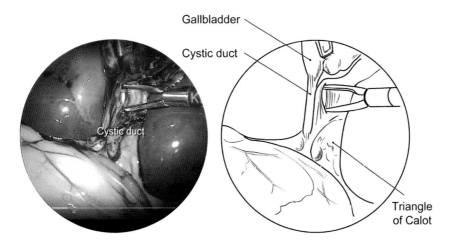

Fig. 148: Photography and videography today are so advanced that they can show medical and scientific processes, structures, and procedures in extraordinary definition (here, a frame from a video on laparoscopic cholecystectomy, or removal of the gallbladder). Medical illustration does not have to be as faithful to reality as a photograph, or try to explain it (*right*).

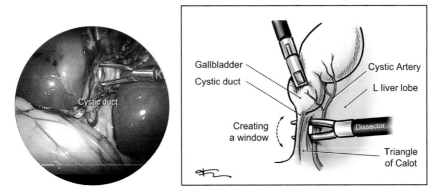

Fig. 149: Instead of tracing a faithful, photographic reproduction, as in Fig. 148, a medical illustrator can reimagine reality to better explain medicine and science.

Chapter 7

The Physician as Visual Communicator

Medical illustration aims to explain a concept, a biochemical cascade, an operation in a way that words alone cannot. The image itself has a didactic value, but so does the *process* to get to the final product. Why did the illustrators choose a particular point of view? Why did they pick specific steps in describing an operation? How did they settle on particular details while omitting others? When we, as viewers, ask ourselves these questions, we become a better, smarter audience. We are no longer passive consumers, and the artist isn't just relying on our collective experience to fill in the missing elements or hidden meanings of a picture. By understanding the creative process, we can meet the artist halfway and reduce these gaps. The universal language Christoph Niemann speaks of (see chapter 5) explains why illustrators do what they do, but we can speak that language too. Not only does medical illustration enhance communication, *understanding* medical illustration makes us better communicators.

Reverse Engineering

As is clear by now, the artistic aspect, while it is the most obvious and often the most stunning part of a medical illustration, is by no means the only one that counts. Even if you have never held a brush in your life, you can apply yourself to scientific visualization. We will not all become great graphic artists, but it can be argued that all doctors draw, and there is nothing wrong with trying to become a little better at it. Furthermore, the skills of a medical illustrator can be useful in many activities of our professional life that do not necessarily rely on images. Deconstructing the process by which a medical illustrator, in collaboration with a clinician or scientist, came to develop the perfect illustration—say, of a novel operation—alerts us to where the crucial steps are, and where we may need to pause. Looking at the perfect illustration of an intracellular process, we are drawn to portions that are highlighted for a reason: that's where the main action is for the topic at hand. If a biochemical cascade flows naturally from top to bottom or from left to right, we need to realize that that is not how it happens in nature; rather, the illustrator made it so after painstaking research into the topic. First, he or she had to understand it, cut through the noise, and plan its visual representation. If we reverse-engineer that thought process, we can better understand the concept itself. And by emulating the illustrator, we, too, can learn how to better communicate in a logical, intuitive fashion.

Physician-educators are not satisfied to merely understand these things; they need to teach them to students, residents, junior colleagues, and peers. Thinking like a medical illustrator can help organize one's thoughts. It starts with the equivalent of the sketch: What is my angle? Which point of view do I want to emphasize? How much detail do I need to provide to make the concept clear, and how much clutter can I safely omit while making the illustration still understandable? Does the narrative flow logically? Scientific communication and medical illustration emphasize the action, the process. Once the initial concept has been sketched, the progression must be thought out. For a surgical intervention, these are the individual and successive steps—from initial incision to optimal exposure of the target organ, from the isolation of crucial blood vessels to the safe resection of the tumor. For a scientific paper, it is the preestablished sequence of the manuscript's sections: Background and Rationale, Methods, Results, Discussion, and Conclusions. A research grant follows the same pattern (the Discussion section having been replaced with Anticipated Results), and clarity is particularly crucial if the investigator hopes to win over the reviewers.

Grantsmanship is more important than ever as more researchers vie for ever-shrinking funding. Not only should the science behind a grant application be flawless, the execution should be crisp, engaging, even riveting. It may be science, but it is still a narrative, writes Josh Ettinger in *Nature,* and Hollywood can teach researchers a lot about scientific storytelling.[1] As I was once told by a colleague who himself reviewed grants for the National Institutes of Health (NIH):

"The proposal must make sense, even at 10,000 feet altitude and with a whiskey in one hand," referring to the fact that many reviewers, like many of us, tend to put off tasks until the last minute, and that their first read of your proposal may well be on a flight to the meeting of the study section. (This is a variant of the elevator pitch mentioned in chapter 5.) While a research paper or a grant application has occasional figures, it may be difficult to see the link between scientific writing and medical illustration. Yet it is all about analytic thinking, organizing one's thoughts, and communicating them clearly—in other words, visualizing ideas.

In the Venn diagram of medical communication, the worlds of graphic visualization and science writing overlap in the area of the slide presentation and its printed form, the scientific poster. It is certainly no coincidence that the department of medical illustration in many a medical school or academic hospital also provides help to make the perfect slides and posters, whether for lectures and classes or medical conferences. By definition, a PowerPoint slide is an information graphic, a visual representation of data. Even when they lack pictures, good slide presentations obey the basic rules of scientific illustration: limited details to avoid information clutter (bullet points, rather than paragraphs of text); esthetics (choice of fonts and colors); and focal points of the illustration (emphasized text, top-to-bottom/ left-to-right readability).

If the principles of a good medical illustration apply to an effective scientific or medical slide, so do the principles of a good narrative. It is not merely sufficient to choose the perfect point of view and the right amount of detail. When describing a process or an operation, selecting the right moments from a continuous time line is crucial, as is the transition between these points in time or space. Just like a well-edited movie, narrating a medical concept must flow naturally and intuitively: viewers do not even realize that the story is not a continuous time line but is instead made up of individual "scenes."[2] They must receive the right amount of detailed information about each step, while never losing track of the long view. In chapter 6, the principles of a logical narrative, which count on the audience to fill in the gaps, were applied to a series of medical illustrations describing a laparoscopic appendectomy (Fig. 142 and Fig. 144). The same is applicable to a lecture: not just one slide but the entire slide presentation. It is not enough to read from top to bottom or from left to right. The progression of the reader's attention on a single page or slide occurs in 2-D, but a time line is unidimensional; at once simple (slide 2 follows slide 1, no questions asked) and limiting, if one needs to present simultaneous processes or switch from detail to overview. A remedy to this linear approach to a narrative is Prezi, and similar Web-based presentation apps: platforms that allows one to show a bird's-eye view of the topic, drill down to details, zoom back out to an overview of the lecture, and alternate easily between the two, the better to contextualize the various elements of a complex presentation. While this type of presentation enjoyed some success, it never really took off beyond the novelty of showing actual deep dives into a topic's various elements. To quote Jim Harvey, "Crap presenters will still present badly with Prezi."[3]

The use of icons and other symbols that are useful shortcuts in graphic designs (see chapter 5) are equally applicable to presentations, whether to indicate motion or passage of time with arrows, or choose the appropriate pictogram or icon to stand in for a broader concept (a building with a red cross is a hospital; a slice of pizza can represent fatty food); these tools are all available to us, whether we are committed to medical illustration or not.

Some medical illustrators, like www.pictureasportal.com's Betsy Palay and Tami Tolpa, have even made a career out of teaching clinicians and scientists how to better present their research, well aware that it is not enough to have a great idea—it is crucially important to know how to sell it.[4] In these tutorials, it is not about the illustration per se: it is all about judicious choice of layout, color, emphasis, and readability.

The Doctor-Patient Relationship

We think of medical presentations mainly in terms of medical education, but it's also about patient education: How do we explain things to patients and their families? Whether we merely talk, or use a whiteboard, pamphlets, or actual slides, well-organized thoughts are important. Images, even rudimentary ones, can help a patient visualize and understand a disease or its treatment much more clearly than medical jargon. And, in an increasingly diverse and multilingual world, images from infographics to full-color illustrations or photographs can transcend language barriers.

Cholecystectomy, the surgical removal of a gallbladder, is one of the most commonly performed operations in the United States. It is typically offered as treatment for gallstones, which cause intermittent abdominal pain, usually after a fatty meal (chronic calculous cholecystitis). Recommending a cholecystectomy implies a relationship of trust with the patient, who will literally place his or her life in the hands of the operating team. One of the best ways to establish that trust is for the patient to understand what the disease process is, why the planned intervention will help, and why the treatment won't cause additional problems; without knowledge of the underlying anatomy and physiology, it would be legitimate to ask how one can live without a gallbladder. After all, doesn't every organ have a purpose?

One of the first rules of good scientific illustration is to know your audience. Who is the illustration intended for? Medical specialists, students, the public at large? When communicating with a patient, similar questions need to be asked. Some patients want to know everything and feel more at ease if they understand the detailed theory behind a disease or a treatment. Others would prefer to get the ten-thousand-foot view or a succinct summary of what it is and what must be done about it. Explaining where gallstones come from, what bile is and what it does, is not an easy task, and illustrations can clearly help. Fig. 150 summarizes a highly simplified version of the relationships between organs, hormones, and pathways that predispose one to stone formation. On its face, the graphic respects most of the tenets of a good medical illustration: intuitive anatomic orientation (liver is up, bladder is down); use of contrast and color to distinguish the pathways (breakdown of red blood cells into biliverdin is mirrored by a red-to-green-fading arrow; a brown arrow represents stercobilin in stools and a yellow one the urobilin in urine); minimal text, and creative use of symbols (serpentine arrow follows the tortuous small bowel loops). Fig. 150 does not make bile metabolism look simple, however. Sometimes a picture is *not* worth a thousand words or, more precisely, a pretty picture may be more confusing than a well-designed diagram. The approach to either, however, should be similar: organize your thoughts, plan a sketch, know your audience.

When gallstones develop in the gallbladder, it is usually due to a breakdown of the delicate compositional balance of bile. Bile may appear as a homogeneous, fluorescent green viscous liquid that tastes horrible, but it is a complex fluid whose components are in a soluble state only when their respective concentrations remain within a narrow range. Bile acids (predominantly cholic acid and chenodeoxycholic acid) are produced by the liver and conjugate with taurine and glycine to form bile salts.[5] The main function of bile and bile salts is to form micelles with fat droplets, microscopic structures that enrobe fat to make it water-soluble, thereby allowing its absorption by the gut. Without bile, we would not be able to absorb and metabolize essential fats, or any of the fat-soluble vitamins (vitamin A, D, E, and

K). A simplified analogy is the effect of dishwashing soap that makes grease water-soluble, and thus washable (or, in our case, digestible). While a kitchen metaphor may seem out of place in a discussion about diseases, remember that referencing known situations to describe

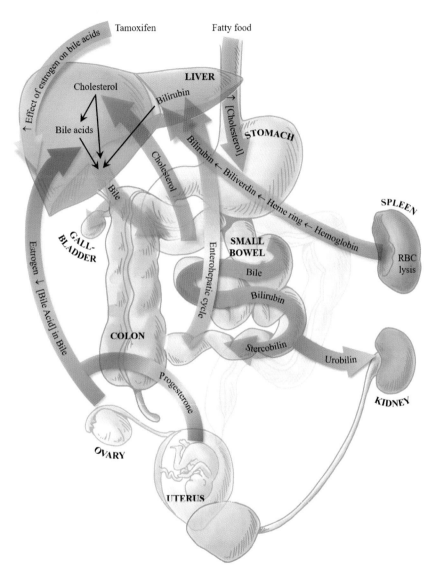

Fig. 150: Bile metabolism. Simplified graph of the various components of bile, the factors that increase or decrease their concentrations, and the pathways of bile secretion and reabsorption. The role of each organ is represented semischematically (approximate anatomic relationships). For example, bile (lime-green arrows) flows from the liver into the gallbladder, where it is stored, and into the duodenum (first portion of the small bowel). Through the action of bacteria, bile is converted in stercobilin, which is excreted in the stools, and urobilin, which is absorbed and excreted in the urine. Bilirubin is also reabsorbed in the last portion of the small bowel and returned to the liver in what is known as the enterohepatic cycle.

hitherto unknown concepts is how we all acquire new knowledge, and medical illustration, specifically, is rife with such examples: think of the "leaves on a bow" used to describe microscopic muscle fibers; monks' cells to describe, well, cells; or the spikes on the wall of the COVID-19 virus that look like rock candy lollipops (chapter 4).

Bile also contains the degradation products of hemoglobin, the macromolecule that gives red blood cells their color and allows transport of oxygen from the lungs to the peripheral tissues (see Fig. 147). When old, damaged, or abnormal red blood cells are destroyed, hemoglobin is released into the bloodstream. Hemoglobin is broken down and the heme rings—the binding sites for oxygen within a hemoglobin molecule—are metabolized into biliverdin, and from there into bilirubin. Bilirubin is excreted in bile and is further transformed once it makes it into the intestinal tract. Downstream degradation leads to stercobilin through bacterial action (this is what gives stools their brown color); and to urobilin, which is absorbed back into the bloodstream and filtered in the urine (urobilin gives urine its yellow color). A higher-than-normal load of bilirubin (for example, because the body breaks down red blood cells at a much higher rate, as in sickle-cell anemia, thalassemia, and hereditary spherocytosis) will increase its concentration in bile, where it will bond with calcium and precipitate as pigment stones. (Here is a second kitchen analogy that may resonate with nonmedical people: one way to explain precipitation and sedimentation, the first steps to stone formation, is to refer to creamy Italian salad dressing. Shake the bottle, and the dressing is homogeneous; let it sit on the countertop for a while, and the silky liquid will start to separate—the olive oil on top, the vinegar below it, and the spices and peppercorns at the bottom. While it is not necessarily an accurate explanation of cholelithiasis, the imagery is clearly understood by most.)

Gallstones form when the many components of bile are out of balance, and biliary pathology is the topic of many a scholarly work. Obviously, most patients may not be too interested in a comprehensive lecture on bile metabolism (and the above description is an abbreviated oversimplification). They are more curious about why *they* have stones, and what can be done about it. Finding a good explanation for the presence of gallstones can be extremely important, even for the less inquisitive person. Is the condition the result of a certain behavior, like diet or contraception? Is it genetic, and is it likely to be passed on to one's offspring? Gallstones are much more common in women than in men. The reasons for this are not completely understood, but women seem predisposed because of an increased synthesis of cholesterol, or an effect of estrogen on bile acids. Pregnancy is associated with a rise in estrogen, progesterone, and other hormones that interact with bile acids; tamoxifen, a hormonal agent active against some types of breast cancer, also affects estrogen metabolism and significantly increases the risk of gallstones. Obesity is associated with an increase in cholesterol synthesis, but rapid weight loss can be a risk factor, too, by inhibiting the secretion of bile acids even more than that of cholesterol. All these factors—behavioral and genetic—affect the risk of cholesterol stones, the most common etiology of gallstones. Biliary excretion of phospholipids (molecules that also help stabilize fat) is impaired in some genetic disorders, which may be more prevalent in certain ethnic groups than others. Even in the absence of disease, the normal concentration of all these components may be genetically determined. Thus, a family history of gallstones may be a strong indicator of whether one develops stones too. The classic representation of this delicate bile solubility balance is a triangle that plots the concentrations of three bile components: cholesterol, phospholipids, and bile salts (Fig. 151).[6] Too much cholesterol or too little bile salts and/or phospholipids results in supersaturation of bile with cholesterol, leading to precipitation and formation of cholesterol stones.[7]

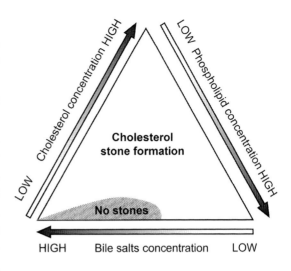

Fig. 151: The bile triangle proposed by William H. Admirand and Donald M. Small. For bile to stay homogeneous and soluble, the concentrations of its components must remain within a narrow window (*gray area at bottom left*): relatively low concentrations of cholesterol and high concentrations of bile salts and phospholipids.

The bile triangle is an elegant and iconic representation of why gallstones form. The illustration itself has endured because of its simplicity: when Admirand and Small reported their study in 1968, they needed to represent the individual concentrations of three key bile components from ninety-one individual patients (sixty-six of whom had gallstones).[8] Scattergrams typically plot out one or two variables at a time and use a classic *XY*-axis graph. Simultaneously representing three intertwined variables is more difficult and would probably generate a more complex, three-dimensional graph, with *X, Y,* and *Z* axes. Clearly, a triangle is easier to draw, and that simple image has been used to explain the formation of gallstones for decades. It is a great mnemonic for medical students and trainees; it is also a useful visual aid for clinicians when they communicate with patients: a simple-to-draw geometric shape can explain how gallstones form without the need for a lengthy biochemical dissertation on lipids, bile salts, and

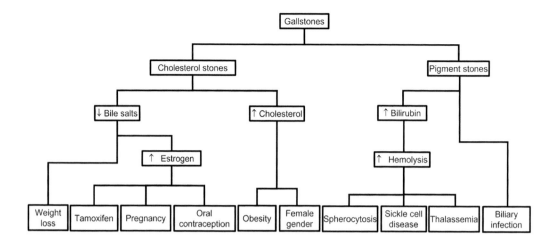

Fig. 152: Differential diagnosis of gallstones. The two most common forms of stones are cholesterol stones (*left*) and pigment stones (*right*). The various causes of stones are organized by pathophysiology, and all possible etiologies are displayed at the bottom.

proteins. The visual aid also helps physicians organize their thoughts: the key elements are cholesterol (a word everyone is familiar with), bile salts, and phospholipids; bile contains all three of these elements; too much of one or two little of another leads to stone formation.

This approach may show *how* stones form, but it does not explain *why* they do. It does not tell patients whether it is something they did, or whether they were born with that risk. It behooves a doctor to understand why a particular condition develops and communicate this to a patient. Fig. 152 summarizes the earlier wordy exposé on all the various causes of cholelithiasis. At the top, the discovery of stones in the gallbladder prompts two pathways: cholesterol stones, by far the most common, and pigment stones, which reflect either a biliary infection (rare, if out of the blue) or an excess bilirubin load due to a hemolytic disease, whereby red blood cells are being destroyed at a fast rate.

The chart is easy to follow, from a single box at the top to the various underlying conditions, and even if it is not as thorough and complete as entire paragraphs, it is comprehensive and logically organized. It reads naturally, from top to bottom, at least for a student who wants to have an overview of the disease, or a clinician who does not yet know what caused the condition in a particular patient: the graph is a clear display of the differential diagnosis, which must be broad enough so nothing gets missed until the clinician narrows it down to only a few, and ultimately a single explanation.

Form must follow purpose, however, and it is important to know the audience. To patients, it matters little what all the various forms of biliary disease are. They want to know what is happening to *them*. Flipping the graph upside down can make more sense (Fig. 153): when the etiology appears straightforward (for example, a young boy whose

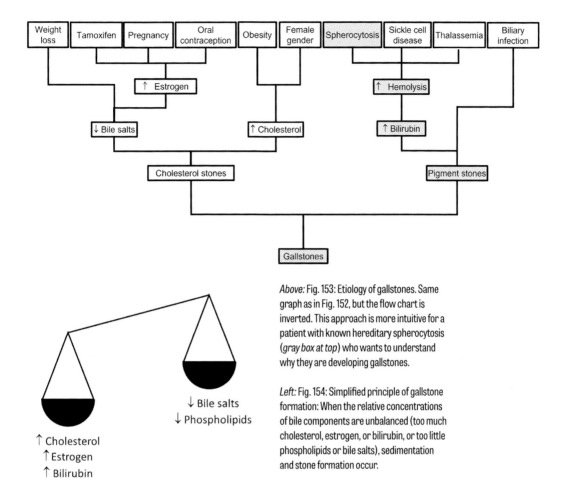

Above: Fig. 153: Etiology of gallstones. Same graph as in Fig. 152, but the flow chart is inverted. This approach is more intuitive for a patient with known hereditary spherocytosis (*gray box at top*) who wants to understand why they are developing gallstones.

Left: Fig. 154: Simplified principle of gallstone formation: When the relative concentrations of bile components are unbalanced (too much cholesterol, estrogen, or bilirubin, or too little phospholipids or bile salts), sedimentation and stone formation occur.

father is known to have spherocytosis, or a woman who just gave birth), a patient may become more engaged if one starts with the most likely underlying condition, and explains (top to bottom) how this caused cholelithiasis. Just like the perfect illustration, the perfect diagram or the perfect explanation must be clear and the progression logical. Patient communication benefits a lot from carefully executed visualization, but it does not always have to be a picture. Oversimplification is not necessarily a bad thing either: the bile triangle (Fig. 151), which is specific to cholesterol stones, and the more detailed diagram (Fig. 153) can be combined into a simple scale of too much of one thing, too little of another that summarizes all types of gallstones (Fig. 154).

Patients who are about to undergo an operation may be interested in why they have a disease, but they are even more interested in what will be done to them. Why is it necessary to remove the gallbladder,

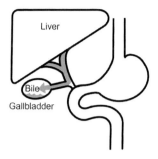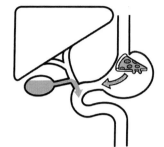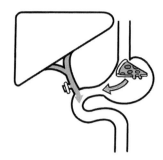

Fig. 155: Schematic representation of bile flow before and after cholecystectomy. *Left:* The liver secretes bile continuously; at rest, most of it is stored in the gallbladder. *Middle:* When we eat a fatty meal (represented by a slice of pizza), the gallbladder contracts and squeezes bile into the intestines to mix with the food. *Right:* After the gallbladder is removed (represented by a clip on the cystic duct), bile continues to flow into the intestines to help digest fat.

and how will they function normally without it? A detailed illustration of the anatomy of the liver, the bile ducts, the gallbladder, and the intestinal tract (like Fig. 6) can be used to demonstrate how the bile is secreted by the liver into the right and left hepatic ducts, which join to form the common hepatic duct; how bile follows the path of least resistance and enters the cystic duct and the gallbladder when the ampulla of Vater is closed. How, triggered by a fatty meal, the sphincter of Oddi, at the junction of the common bile duct, the pancreatic duct, and the duodenum, relaxes at the same time that the gallbladder contracts, squirting a dollop of bile to help digest the food. Some patients may be fascinated by the wonders of human anatomy and physiology, but the anatomic relationships can be whittled down to a minimum without losing the essence: when fasting, bile flows from the liver to the gallbladder; when we eat, the gallbladder empties bile into the intestine to mix with food (Fig. 155). A simple diagram, if well planned, logically reads from top to bottom, aided by directional arrows. The diagram also shows that the main bile ducts, from the liver to the intestines, are untouched by removing the gallbladder, which is connected by a sidetrack. Without a gallbladder, bile continuously drips into the intestines, and fat absorption continues normally.

In all these examples, the concept of medical illustration, or visualization, is not taken literally. Whether the final result is figurative art, a minimalistic drawing, or a chart, planning any form of visual information is a process that helps us understand the problem, analyze its essential aspects, and present them clearly to our audience. Knowing how medical illustrators work not only makes us appreciate their craft, it teaches us to become better communicators. (Write what you know, as the advice goes. The cholecystectomy example may seem oddly specific, but the principle is applicable to any topic one masters and needs to impart to others.)

Medical Comics

Communicating well with patients, students, or peers implies listening. To be effective in our rapport with others, we must understand them and show compassion and empathy. That is certainly the theory behind art appreciation in medical school, and it is also reflected in the know-your-audience tenet of good medical illustration. Classic medical illustration is at its best when it demonstrates concrete concepts: an operative procedure, a cellular cascade, and anatomic relationship. Can visual communication be useful in expressing feelings as well? Certainly, there are plenty of examples in classic paintings, from Frida Kahlo sublimating her chronic pain (Fig. 66) to the feeling of angst, despair, and gloom in Edvard Munch's *The Scream* and *The Inheritance* (Fig. 50). As demonstrated by Holly Quinton, a Newcastle general practice physician and artist, drawings, illustrations, and metaphors can also be used by real-life patients to explain what they experience, from splitting headache to tingling and tinnitus.[9] In general, however, moods and thoughts are more easily expressed in writing: the printed word is a more precise way to convey emotions to an audience. But just as we are not all graphic artists, most of us are not born writers, and expressing one's feelings in long form can be intimidating. Enter medical comics, a relatively new iteration of an older tradition. In chapter 5, the language of comics is mentioned as an inspiration for modern medical illustration, with its visual representation of dynamism and its use of icons and symbols to represent action or movement: sweat beads, dust clouds, lightning bolts, and wisps of smoke. Comics also borrow from cinema to teach us about narrative, moving from frame to frame, just like medical illustrations of a process progress from step to step intuitively.

It is unclear why medical comics became a thing when they did, but their popularity seems to coincide with the recent return-to-humanism-in-medicine phenomenon, itself a reaction to the ever-increasing role that technology plays in our daily lives. Despite its name, a medical comic is not a cartoon about doctors, nor is it a comic book–style pamphlet to entertain children who are about to undergo surgery. It is not the same as a graphic novel about a medical topic, one of the most remarkable examples of which is the Zombie Pandemic project produced by the Centers for Disease Control and Prevention (CDC) in 2011.[10] In response to the flood of inquiries about zombie attacks they received in the wake of popular zombie movies and television series, the CDC developed a campaign—complete with posters and a thirty-six-page full-color graphic novel—to inform the public on how to prepare for the zombie apocalypse. "If you can't beat them, join them," the CDC argued. If the public knew how to prepare for a fictional infestation of undead creatures, they would be ready to face any real emergency, from wildfires to hurricanes.

Preparedness 101: Zombie Pandemic is not really a medical comic. That is not to say that medical comics cannot be fully developed, glossy graphic novels; that they cannot be one-liners, like *New Yorker* cartoons; or that they cannot be directed at younger readers. What unites them is a desire to express feelings, emotions, experiences in a way that is accessible to the reader, who may not want to read a lengthy essay on end-of-life experience, physician burnout, or healthcare disparity. They are accessible to a cancer patient, a discouraged family member, or an overwhelmed nurse who want to express their state of mind without the barriers of a long-form written narrative. The medical comic is a perfect metaphor for the power of medical illustration, and art in general, as a means to communicate, to listen, and to make us more compassionate. Medical comics differ a lot from medical illustration, too: it is not all about efficiency, clarity, compression of time and space, or economy of words. Rather, it is a way to express a mood, a state of mind using two seemingly opposite approaches: text and image. Just like graphic novels and cartoons, medical comics can be text-heavy or wordless, visually beautiful or graphically sober, but the most effective ones get their message across with just the right combination of words and illustrations. The reaction to a good medical comic may not necessarily be "How beautiful," but rather "How very true!"—a sense of connection with the author, a recognition of shared experiences or an epiphany about how "the other half lives."[11]

Some in the medical profession have been prolific producers of medical comics. M. K. (MaryKay) Czerwiec, RN, MA, is a nurse and educator who teaches graphic medicine at the University of Illinois Medical School and the Art Institute of Chicago. She is an artist-in-residence at the Center for Medical Humanities and Bioethics at Northwestern Medical School and a pioneer in medical comics (her Twitter handle is ComicNurse).[12] She is a coauthor of the *Graphic Medicine Manifesto* and speaks out about the role of comics in healthcare. Her work is not limited to her own experience as a nurse, but most of her books deal with medical situations, from caring for HIV patients or assisting the terminally ill to the anxiety of living with protruding ears. Without denigrating ComicNurse's talent in any way, it is fair to say that her comics are not polished illustrations—in fact, many other medical comics utilize little more than stick figures with speech balloons, a

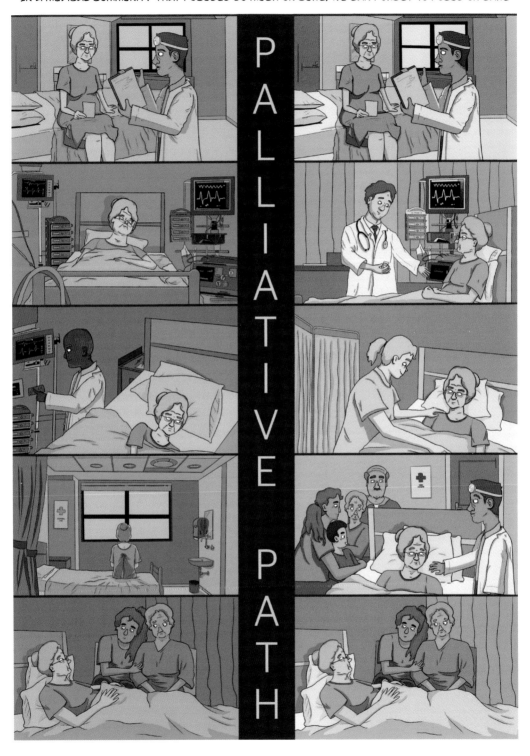

far cry from sophisticated graphic novels or superhero comics, and are sometimes very close to something "my six-year-old could draw." That is often the point, in fact: an accessible, democratic medium that is available to anyone, and allows one to use funny-looking characters to express one's feelings. There are now workshops that help patients voice their anxiety or impotence toward their situation, including in-hospital activities that are part of the increasingly popular healing arts programs.[13] The medical establishment is noticing too. Several specialty journals, like the venerable *Annals of Internal Medicine,* now regularly publish medical comics as part of their monthly online content (free of charge at http://annals.org/graphicmedicine), "bringing together original graphic narratives, comics, animation and other creative forms by those who provide or receive healthcare."[14]

Medical comics are just the latest embodiment of how visual communication improves doctor-patient relationships and makes us more compassionate caregivers. And while it doesn't require one to be an artist, having some graphic talent doesn't hurt. Shirlene Obuobi, MD, is a fellow in cardiology who is also a gifted graphic artist. She is very well known for her spot-on descriptions of the lives of medical students, interns, and senior residents. Medical training is notoriously harsh, and young physicians-to-be must juggle impossibly rough schedules with the emotional stress of caring for sick patients and the insecurities of being a very junior member of the medical team. Dr. Obuobi (@shirlywhirlmd) has clearly touched a nerve, and her comics have garnered a very large following. She is also a vocal advocate for equity and diversity at all levels of the healthcare community, showing once again (see chapter 3) that medical illustration and medical comics can be agents of social change.

Communicating through medical comics should not be hampered by a lack of artistic skills, but a solid foundation in medical illustration can lead to beautiful results. Through a generous grant from the Gold Humanism Honor Society, we have started a pilot project at the Alpert Medical School of Brown University, enrolling students who have taken our medical illustration course into a medical comics workshop. In discussion sessions with facilitators, students develop narratives about personal experiences or observations and build one-page medical comics using some of the principles of medical illustration outlined in the previous chapters while learning the grammar of comics and graphic novels.[15] Fig. 156 shows Frank Deng's interpretation of the role of technology in medicine today, and the ease with which we may lose the personal touch: even when the outcome is hopeless and the course of a disease cannot be altered, the final journey can be made so much more humane when we remember to communicate and take time to be in the moment. The color schemes of two identical time lines, shown vertically side by side, reflect the different approaches: the cold, impersonal, blue-green hues of machines, monitors, and instruments versus the warm orange-red tones of human contact. Ironically, this comic, which was published in *Annals of Internal Medicine*,[16] predates the COVID-19 pandemic, which forced us all to make sometimes heart-wrenching decisions. Even when we wanted to be physically close to our loved ones, we couldn't, and we had to rely on technology, such as tablets and video feeds, to make someone's final days more humane.

Medical illustration is about the story behind the image: organizing one's thoughts, planning a sketch, finding the best way to communicate with our students, our peers, and our patients. Graphs, schematics, and diagrams are all part of visual communication, and they are accessible to all of us. We can even use the concept of visual communication to communicate feelings, to become more empathic and compassionate caregivers.[17] Thus, anyone can be a medical illustrator, as long as we are not asked to illustrate.

Chapter 8

The Physician as Illustrator

Although many scientific illustrations are true works of art, their primary function is to explain, simplify, and synthetize in ways that words alone cannot. A simple black-and-white line drawing can be much more informative than an elaborate full-color painting—it is the ultimate effect that counts. You do not have to be an accomplished artist to get your point across. This is good news for the rest of us, of course. We can all be visual communicators.

As Peter La Fleur says in *Dodgeball,* "You are perfect just the way you are." But if you wouldn't mind getting a little bit better at illustrating, it can't hurt to master a few rudiments of drawing techniques. Not only can it make the end result prettier, it can make the message clearer. Whether it is a quick diagram on a white board, a "napkin sketch," or even a more elaborate figure for a presentation or a manuscript, pen-and-ink can convey a lot of information, and a lot of detail can be rendered using some simple concepts.

Light and Darkness

The overarching goal of any two-dimensional illustration is to give it a three-dimensional impression. To give the illusion of volume and depth, a drawing must overcome the limitation of a flat sheet of a paper, as well as the absence of depth perception by the viewer, which in real life comes from stereoscopic vision—our eyes capture two slightly different images, which, when combined, allows us to see in 3-D. Any

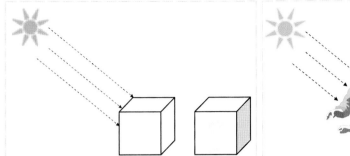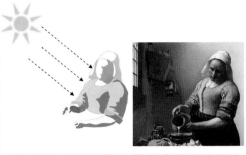

2-D illustration must therefore use "tricks" to render volume to the depicted objects. The most effective way to do this is to reproduce the effect of light and shadow. Subjects with a rich variation in light intensity appear less two-dimensional and are visually more interesting. Brightly lit images are often flatter and less appealing, which is why most nature photographers and painters avoid working at midday, preferring early mornings or late afternoons when the sun is lower and the shadows are longer.

By convention, light comes from the top left (Fig. 157). The portions or sides of a subject closest to that light source will be brighter or lighter, while the areas away from it (bottom right) will be darker. This principle has been documented for millennia and is not limited to illustration: it is found in cartography, portrait photography, computer interfaces, and many other fields. It can be a useful exercise to guess where the light is coming from when looking at paintings or photographs (Fig. 158). Jan Vermeer's paintings are particularly "illuminating" in that regard: often the window, the single source of light, is visible in the painting. Because many of his paintings have one or two dominant characters close to the window, the light-dark distribution can be striking. Even when the window is not visible, in fact, its presence off-screen can be inferred from the location of light and dark areas (Fig. 159). (Note that both Vermeer paintings in Fig. 159 also feature anatomic curios: *Study of a Young Woman* shows the subject staring straight at the painter, and there is something off in her face: her eyes are wide-set, a condition called hypertelorism, sometimes seen with craniosynostosis and other disorders of the skull. Some have pointed out that the subject in *Girl with the Pearl Earring* does not seem to have eyebrows, and have wondered what she is hiding under the head scarf. Could she be suffering from alopecia? This is all speculation, of course, but baldness may have been an acquired and desirable feature in Golden Age Holland. Gianluca Nazzaro argues that a high forehead was a sign of beauty in women, and refers to the practice of plucking one's hair for that

Left: Fig. 157: By convention, light comes from the top left. Surfaces that are away from the light are in the shadow and are therefore darker.

Right: Fig. 158: Example of a figure illuminated by a single light source, *top left* (sunlight coming through the window). The parts that are away from the light lie in the shadows and are therefore darker. Johannes Vermeer, *Het Melkmeisje* (The milkmaid), circa 1660.

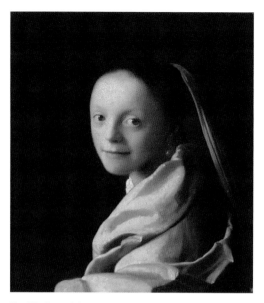
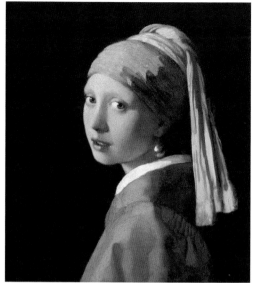
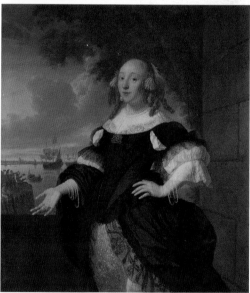

Fig. 159: *Above:* Johannes Vermeer. In both portraits, light seems to come from the left, presumably through a window that is off-stage. These types of portraits, meant as character studies, were popular in seventeenth-century Netherlands, and are referred to as tronies, or *mugs. Above left: Study of a Young Woman,* 1665–67. Although it is not pathognomonic of a specific syndrome, she has wide-set eyes (hypertelorism). *Above right:* Johannes Vermeer's *Meisje met de Parel* (Girl with a pearl earring), 1665, has been noted by some to lack eyebrows, raising the question of alopecia, suggesting that the headscarf hides baldness. Others point to the fad of plucking one's hair to enlarge the forehead, a canon of beauty at the time. *Right:* Bartholomeus van der Helst, *Geertruida den Dubbelde,* 1667, who may represent the beauty canon of the era, complete with hairless forehead.

purpose, resulting in frontal fibrosing alopecia, as seen in some other seventeenth-century Dutch paintings.[1])

The fact that we intuitively assume light comes from above seems logical: the primordial light source is the sun. Why top *left,* though? It has been argued that it is what most people tend to favor, the majority of people being right-handed. While it is fascinating to imagine that right- or left-hand dominance might influence how we see the world, a less prosaic explanation might be that when the light source shines from the top right (whether from natural light through a window, a candle,

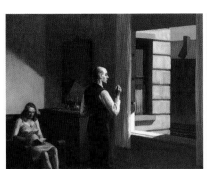
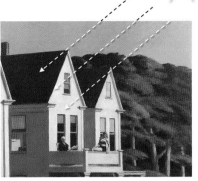

Fig. 160: In many paintings by Edward Hopper, the light comes from the top right, and the darker areas of objects and the objects' shadows are on the left. (*Left: Hotel by a Railroad,* 1952. *Right: Second Story Sunlight,* 1960.)

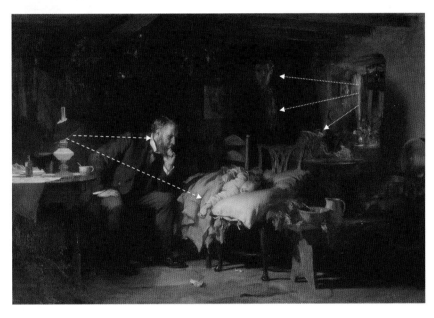

Fig. 161: Multiple light sources (arrows). The focus of the painting is on the doctor and his young patient, both illuminated by the oil lamp on the table (dashed arrows), which suggests he has been watching over her all night, but a second source of light, the dawning day, comes in through a crack in the window (dotted arrows), illuminating the father from the right. Sir Luke Fildes, *The Doctor,* 1891.

or a lamp), the hand of a right-handed artist casts a disturbing shadow on the area that is being drawn. It is therefore easier for a right-handed person to place the light source on the left. One significant weakness in this theory is the fact that the works of many famous left-handed artists, such as Leonardo da Vinci and M. C. Escher, do not tend to show top-right illumination, whereas a large number of paintings by Edward Hopper and Giorgio de Chirico (both known to be right-handed) do (Fig. 160).

Real life is always more complicated, and light can come in from multiple sources (Fig. 161). It also reflects off bright surfaces and mirrors, creating a complex pattern of dark and light hues. However, the

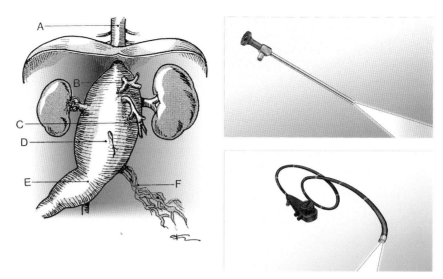

Left: Fig. 162: The eye is drawn toward the brightly lit abdominal aortic aneurysm (D) in the middle of the image, in part because it stands in contrast with the darker retroperitoneal background.

Right: Fig. 163: Light from a rigid telescope (*top*) or flexible endoscope (*bottom*) originates from its tip, creating a visual field that is illuminated head-on from the direction of the viewer.

goal of medical illustration is not to represent real life as faithfully as possible, but to document and explain complex ideas more clearly. As such, the use of light and dark becomes part of a language with its clear and often intuitive rules, allowing the viewer to easily grasp the shapes of objects and organs and situate them in space. Even when a composition may appear "natural" and faithful to life, great artists have in fact used this visual language to highlight or explain particular aspects of their work, drawing the viewer to the focus point of the image. In *The Doctor* painting (Fig. 161), the main action is the attentive physician at the child's bedside; the light from the nightstand illuminates the faces and the white linen, making it the center of attention. The shaft of daylight through the crack in the window is not only an interesting visual effect, illuminating the father, who would otherwise be hidden in the dark background. Sir Luke Fildes himself says that "[It signifies] the imminent recovery of the child."

The use of light and light sources is also an important feature of medical and scientific illustrations, and often for the same reasons: to draw the viewer to the important aspect of the image. In Fig. 162, the background (retroperitoneum) is darker, in contrast with the brightly lit, white abdominal aorta with its aneurysm.

When a medical illustrator captures a natural, lifelike clinical scene, there is very little about it that is, in fact, "natural." Clinical situations are often staged. Whether it is an image seen through a microscope or an endoscope, or a scene in an operating room, the lighting is artificial. Illumination is altered to highlight the focus of the procedure or point of interest, which sometimes obscures the

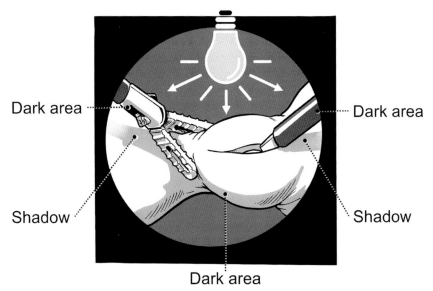

Dark area

Dark area

Shadow

Shadow

Dark area

Fig. 164: Light from a telescope (arrows) originates from the same point as the observer, casting shadows radially in all directions.

natural shadow-and-light conventions that help us see in three dimensions. In endoscopy and laparoscopic (minimally invasive) surgery, for example, the light source comes from the same point in space as the observer (Fig. 163). The objects closest to the lens are therefore brightly illuminated but lack distinctive shadow patterns that would help recognize volumes and perspective. Additionally, the pinpoint light source is so close that the shadows and dark surfaces are cast radially in the periphery of the field of vision rather than in the same direction, for example, toward the bottom right (Fig. 164).

Dinosaur Prints

Without context clues, such as a window through which the sun is shining or a lamp on a table, our brain defaults to the assumption that light is coming from the top left. As stated before, the parts of an object that are the farthest away from the light, or are obstructed from the light source, will be darker. This means that for a convex volume, the darkest area will be at the bottom right. Concave volumes, in contrast, have a darker area closest to the light source (Fig. 165) because the ridge of the concavity closest to the light obstructs its path. The farthest portion of the concavity receives unobstructed beams and is therefore lighter. While Fig. 165 illustrates this in a two-dimensional cross section of convexity and concavity, the same applies to a three-dimensional object. The shape in Fig. 166A is neutral—it is a mere

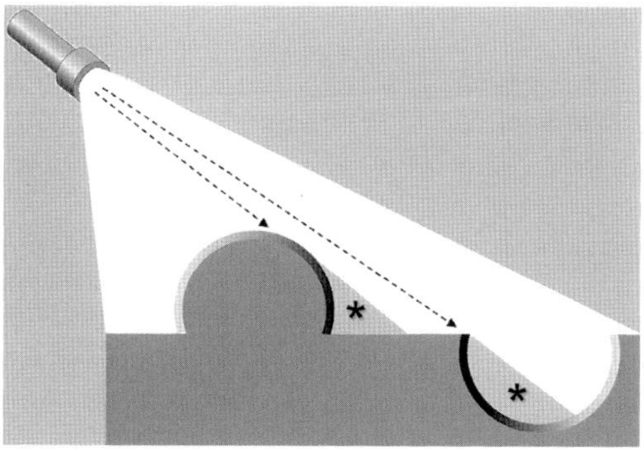

Fig. 165: With convex shapes (*left*), the side closest to the light will be brightly lit, while the side furthest from it will be in the dark (dashed arrows and *). With concave shapes (*right*), the opposite is true: the side closest to the light is obscured by the concavity's ridge,* while the light path is unobstructed away from the light source.

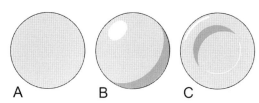

Fig. 166: Conveying volume to a two-dimensional shape by rendering light and dark areas. A circle (A) can be made to look like a sphere (B) by darkening the area furthest from the light (assumed to be top left) and adding a bright spot closest to the light source. Darkening an area closest to the light source, in contrast, will suggest a concave structure, such as a normal, biconcave red blood cell (C).

A   B   C

circle. To convey convexity—that is, to describe a sphere—the area away from the light source must be darker (Fig. 166B). Conversely, shading the area closest to the light will give the impression of a concave volume (Fig. 166C).

A perfect medical illustration of this can be found in hematology: the difference between a normal red blood cell, which is a biconcave disc (see Fig. 147), and an abnormal (spherical) red blood cell seen in hereditary spherocytosis. (The phylogenetic significance of a biconcave red blood cell may lie in its function. The most evolutionary effective oxygen carrier cell is one that has the greatest surface area for a given volume, allowing efficient transmembrane passage of oxygen into the cytoplasm, where it is bound to hemoglobin. That ratio is the smallest for a perfect sphere, and greater for biconcave structures.)

While the example of red blood cells seems unique, the depiction of concavities is omnipresent: The cross section of hollow structures, such as blood vessels or intestinal loops, are nothing more than concavities, and using the light-and-dark conventions to depict them is a simple and effective way to bring an illustration to life. So engrained in our brain is the concept of "light from above" that we automatically see convexity or concavity in a volume based on the distribution of light and dark areas. Consider the fossils in the Dinosaur Footprints Reservation in Holyoke, Massachusetts. Approximately two hundred million years ago, dinosaurs roaming the then mudflats of that area left footprints in the soft mud, which then dried up. Come the next

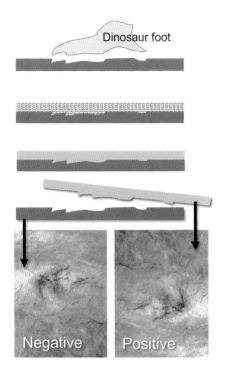

Dinosaur foot

Dinosaur makes a print in the ground

Mud fills up the print holes

Mud petrifies

Layers of rock are carefully separated
– leaving positive and negative print
fossils

Negative   Positive

Fig. 167: Formation
of fossilized
dinosaur prints in
the Patriot Valley,
Massachusetts.
As the mud filling
the holes petrified,
positive and
negative prints
were formed.

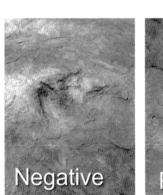

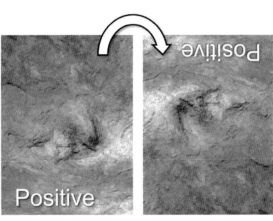

Negative   Positive   ǝʌᴉʇᴉsoԀ

Fig. 168: The two
photographs in
Fig. 167 are, in
fact, identical, but
turning a concave
print upside
down makes it
appear convex, so
engrained is our
notion that light
on top and dark at
the bottom suggest
convexity.

rainy season, the holes filled up with another layer of mud (Fig. 167).
These successive strata of mud eventually petrified, but the layers of
stone can be carefully separated. This produces a series of negative
footprints (the actual imprint of the dinosaur's feet), and their positive
counterparts: raised structures resembling the dinosaurs' soles. Without situational clues (either stereoscopic vision, or a clear indication
of where the light is coming from), it can be assumed that the prints
whose dark areas are at the bottom right are convex (positive prints),
while those with dark areas at the top left are concave (negative). Fig.
168 reveals the trickery of light and shadow: the same 2-D photograph

of a print can be made to look concave or convex, depending on the position of light and dark areas.

In didactic medical illustrations—as opposed to realistic paintings, or art for art's sake—it is important to respect these conventions. While it may be an oversimplification of the subject that is being illustrated, clear separation between light and dark, and consistent use of the top-left illumination principle make the illustration easier to understand. (If there is a good reason to deviate from the top-left illumination, as with laparoscopy, for example Fig. 164, the position of the light source should be made clear.)

Shadows

Not only do volumes have lighter and darker areas when properly illuminated, they also cast shadows. Drawing the shadow of an object or organ might sound like a frivolous move but, just as light and dark areas of an object give us clues as to its volume, shadows add information about the relationships between organs or structures. Shadows are created by obstruction of the light beams by an object. A few simplified (even if not always completely accurate) rules can help us utilize an object's shadow to improve the clarity of the illustration. The taller an object, the longer the shadow it casts. In Fig. 169, the two columns are obviously of uneven lengths, and their shadows are different as well. But note that even in a top-down view (inset), which does not show the actual height of each column, their respective shadows give it away.

Shadows tell us something about the shape and size of the object. They also tell us something about the surface below the object. Shadows are sharpest and most visible on smooth, light surfaces. Darker,

Left: Fig. 169: The taller an object (or the lower the light source, as when the sun is setting), the longer the shadow. When illustrating two similar objects with different heights, showing a difference in shadows can enhance the 3-D effect.

Right: Fig. 170: In general, when an object is not touching the underlying surface, its shadow doesn't touch the object either (*right*). (Note also that the shadow cast by an object is larger and fainter when it is farther away from its underlying surface, as with the ball on the right.)

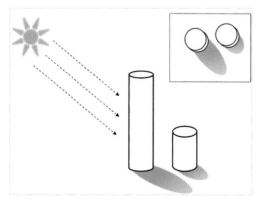

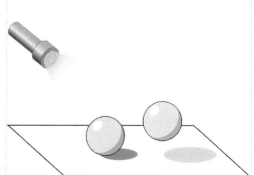

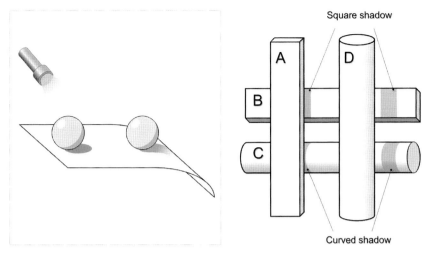

Square shadow

A   D

B

C

Curved shadow

Left: Fig. 171: The shape of a shadow is determined by the shape of its object, as well as by the shape of the underlying surface. On the right, the downward curve of the plane causes the sphere's shadow to be elongated.

Right: Fig. 172: Relationship between objects, as reflected by their shadows. A is touching B and C, hence A and its shadows touch; B is a flat surface, and A's shadow is therefore straight; C is curved, and A's shadow on it is therefore curved as well (and shortest in the middle, where A and C are in contact). D stands in front of A and doesn't touch B or C; the shadows cast on B and C therefore don't touch D.

rough, or fuzzy surfaces produce less obvious shadows, as do reflective surfaces.

As a rule, if an object touches the surface it stands on, the shadow will touch the object as well (Fig. 170). If an object does not touch the surface below it, the shadow will *usually* not touch the object either. This phenomenon can be used very effectively to illustrate the position of an object or organ in space, relative to its landmarks. (Because of the radial direction of the light beams, particularly for a close-by light source, the shadow will also appear larger the farther the object is from the surface; and because of ambient light reflecting off other objects and surfaces, the shadow will be progressively lighter and less defined the farther an object is from the surface.)

In the examples above, we were mostly concerned with the object itself, assuming that the surface it sits on is flat. However, the shape of the shadow is also determined by the shape (not just the position) of the underlying surface. Mastering the deformation of a shadow based on the shape of the underlying surface can be difficult, but some basic concepts are relatively simple: since the shadow is smaller when an object touches the surface, a surface that is curved *away* from the object will show a larger shadow (or portion thereof). In the example in Fig. 171, the ball on the right sits on a surface that is curving downward, away from the ball, and its shadow is therefore elongated. Fig. 172 summarizes all the effects described above: Object A is touching B and C, and its shadows are therefore touching object A as well. Because C has a curved surface, the areas that are not in contact with A have a curved shadow. D is also in front of B and C, but the fact that its shadows, both straight and curved, are shown away from D suggests that D is well in front of

B and C without touching them. Thus, D stands in the foreground; A stands behind D, but in front of B and C.

The judicious distribution of dark and light areas, and the placement of shadows, can give a tridimensional appearance to the simplest of drawings. It can indicate whether objects (or parts of them) are convex or concave; whether they are touching or not; and whether the undersurface is flat, convex, or concave. It can be a helpful exercise to examine seemingly more complex illustrations, and search for

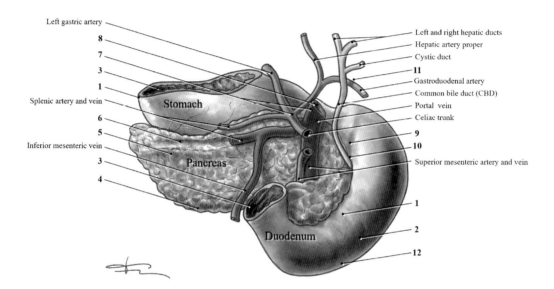

Fig. 173: Simple principles of light and dark, shadows, convexity, and concavity can be found in more complex illustrations as well—here, a posterior view of the pancreas, the stomach, and the duodenum. 1: The stomach and duodenum are convex organs, and the parts closest to the top-left illumination source are lighter. 2: The parts of the organs away from the light are darkest. 3: They are hollow organs, and their lumen is concave—the top-left light illuminates the right side of the concavity, while the part closest to the light source is darker. 4: The edges of the pancreas are slightly rounded (convex), shown by the darker bottom part. 5: The organ itself is not round like the duodenum, and is in fact a little scalloped, as indicated by a slight concavity at the top, which is a little darker than the uniformly shaded body of the pancreas. 6: The splenic vein runs posterior to the pancreas and lies in a groove; that concave groove is illustrated by a darker area on top. 7: Blood vessels are cylinders—externally convex—hence the lighter area at left (closest to the light source). Arteries are true cylinders, while veins are thin-walled and more collapsible: they have a flattened, slightly concave wall, demonstrated by the darker portion of the portal vein closest to the light. 8: Blood vessels are hollow, and their cut surface is therefore concave (darkest part is closest to the light source). 9: The common bile duct runs well posteriorly to the duodenum (in this view from behind; *posterior* means closer to the viewer), and the shadow it casts on the duodenum doesn't touch the duct. 10: At its most distal end, it joins the duodenum, touching it, and the duct and its shadow converge as well. 11: The gastroduodenal artery runs anterior to the common bile duct without touching it, as suggested by the off-set position of the duct's shadow on the artery. 12: Although there is a dominant light source (intuitively placed top left), ambient light and bright surfaces cause some light to be reflected at the far-right edges of three-dimensional structures. This "halo" gives the illustration a more realistic appearance.

manifestations of these principles. Fig. 173 is such an illustration, and while it is intricate and shows much more detail than the examples earlier in this chapter, the principles remain the same.

Pen Lines and Texturing

Conveying a palpable volume to a two-dimensional painting is all about illumination, shadows, and light, and the use of colors or gray scales. Drawing and sketching don't pretend to be photo-realistic. Instead, pen-and-ink, black-and-white illustrators must *signal* three dimensions with the few tools at their disposal: line thickness, high contrasts, and judicious utilization of white spaces and texturing.

The simple combination of thick and thin lines can substantially increase the volume of a pen drawing in several ways. To better define an object, a volume, a structure, or an organ, its outline can be made thicker than its inner details (Fig. 174). Even without adding shading, coloring, or texturing, the thick contour clearly delineates the object and separates it from its surroundings.

Line thickness can also be used to replace shading of the volume and suggest illumination. Instead of darkening the part of a volume that is away from the light source (see Fig. 157), the dark side of the object's contour can be thickened (Fig. 174). Fig. 174 also illustrates a technique that combines contour lines and shadow rendering: rather than using a uniform line thickness, the areas where structures meet, bend, fold, or crease are accentuated with a curvi-triangular black area (in the line drawing of the fetus in Fig. 174, these black accents

Fig. 174: Thicker lines define the contours of an object or organ, make it stand out and give it more volume. Thinner lines can be used for inner details. Line thickness can also be used instead of shading: in the illustration of the fetus (*right*), the outline of the back and other parts away from a top-left light source are thicker. Where body parts cross, the shadows they cast on each other are suggested by triangular-shaped black areas, a technique called *snodgrassing*.

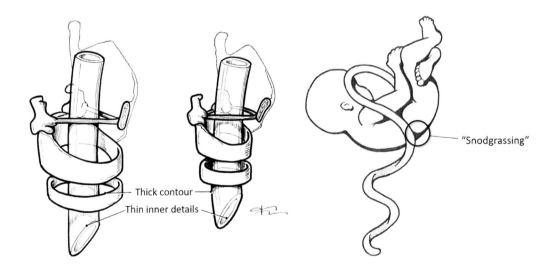

Thick contour
Thin inner details

"Snodgrassing"

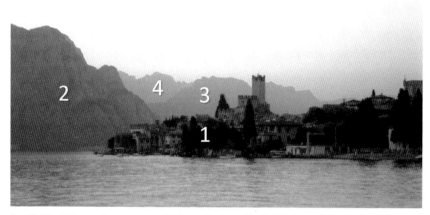

Fig. 175: Objects that are far away appear lighter and hazier, as light is absorbed by the atmosphere. *Above:* View of Scaligero Castle in Malcesine, on Lake Garda, Italy, in the foreground (1). The mountain ranges in the background (2–4) are progressively hazier as they are farther away from the viewer.

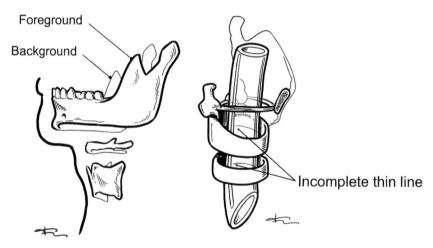

Left: This effect can be reproduced by using thinner lines to draw the right wings of the hyoid and thyroid cartilages and the right ramus of the mandible. Their left counterparts have thicker contours, indicating that they are closer. *Right:* Fig. 176: Conveying transparency in line drawings. The endotracheal tube is semiopaque, and the anatomic structures behind it can be faintly seen in transparency, indicated by thin contour lines of the left arytenoid cartilage and the far portion of the tracheal rings. These transparency lines are interrupted (arrows) by two fine vertical lines on the tube, close to its left-sided edge, representing the light reflection on the tube.

are seen as the umbilical cord crosses the eyebrow, the left foot lies over the right thigh, and the right arm casts shadows on the fetus's abdomen and leg). This technique is called *snodgrassing* after the entomologist and illustrator Robert E. Snodgrass.[2] Snodgrassing is also seen in Fig. 174 (at the corners of the endotracheal tube and the overlying tracheal rings) and in Fig. 178 (where the lower lip touches

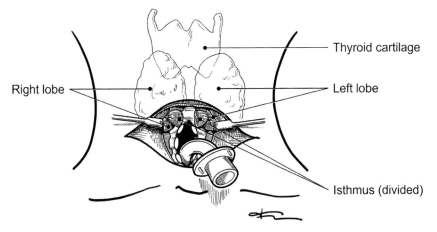

Right lobe

Thyroid cartilage

Left lobe

Isthmus (divided)

Fig. 177: Illustration of tracheostomy. Through the incision, the lower portion of both thyroid lobes and divided isthmus can be seen. The rest of the gland is obscured by the anterior neck wall, but is projected (with thin, interrupted lines) as if the skin were transparent.

the tape). It is an effective "trick"—and the word itself pleasantly rolls off the tongue.

Differential line thickness can suggest depth and distance. The laws of perspective drawing (horizon, vanishing points, orthogonal lines) can be daunting to the incidental illustrator, but simple techniques can go a long way without the need for an elaborate rule book. The farther an object is, the smaller it appears and the hazier it looks. Because sunlight is absorbed by the atmosphere, faraway structures seem grayer and lighter until they completely fade into the background sky. Similarly, structures that are farther away can be drawn with thinner lines, while those in the foreground have thicker contours (Fig. 175).

Finally, thin lines can also be used to convey transparency. Structures can be faintly seen behind semiopaque or transparent objects, such as the endotracheal tube shown in Fig. 176. This transparency effect can be further enhanced by drawing an incomplete thin line. In Fig. 176, the lower border of the first tracheal ring is shown as a thin line as it courses behind the endotracheal tube, but the light reflection on the tube masks the leftmost portion of that line. Drawing an incomplete line can strengthen the sensation of semitransparency. In another example of how drawing conventions have become part of our visual vocabulary, transparency can be suggested with thin, interrupted lines even when the surface of an object is opaque. This is the case in Fig. 177, where the thyroid cartilage and thyroid gland are projected on the obviously opaque skin of the anterior neck. The major portion of each thyroid lobe is hidden, except for the lower aspects, visible in thicker lines inside the wound.

Surface rendering of three-dimensional structures and organs, such as the anatomy of the pancreas in Fig. 173 and the red blood cell

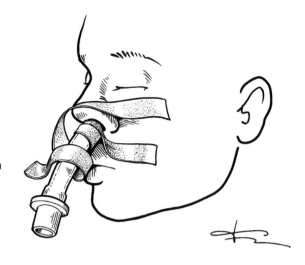

Fig. 178: Line drawing of the proper technique to secure a nasotracheal tube. Instead of detailed shading or coloring, the shadows and darker portions of the illustration are rendered with a few cross-hatching lines and dots. All lighter portions of the image are left white, but the outlines and judicious texturing are enough to give an impression of volume.

pathway in Fig. 147, can be time-consuming and not worth many clinicians' time. Full-color or grayscale illustrations can also be difficult to reproduce, whether in original print or in photocopies. The time-honored crafts of woodcuts and copper engravings, and the tradition of caricatures and cartoons can help us simplify illustrations while conveying a sense of volume, density, and texture. Various techniques of texturing exist and can be used in combination to further enrich an illustration. Most assume a high-contrast environment, where everything that is somewhat light in color or shade is shown as white.

The child in Fig. 178 is clearly not albino or terminally anemic. We understand that the large white surface that is his face is not really white—it is just pale enough that we need only a contour line to understand the surface. Where we need to indicate shadows or volume, a few extra lines suffice, like the dark side of the nose bridge or the shadow cast by the piece of tape over the left nostril. While a more elaborate sketch would involve shading in every aspect that is not pure white, it would not likely make it clearer. This idea is masterfully demonstrated in three almost identical illustrations by Max Brödel, shown in Fig. 179.

The grayscale carbon dust painting of the kidney at the left is particularly realistic, while the pen-and-ink drawing on the right reduces the renal tissues to a mere outline. Although the kidney appears white, the viewer knows not to take that literally.

Used sparingly, texturing adds to the depth and richness of a black-and-white illustration (Fig. 180). The oldest form of texturing in print is the woodcut, a classic style recognizable by its tapered parallel lines that are attached to the perpendicular contour line of the object.

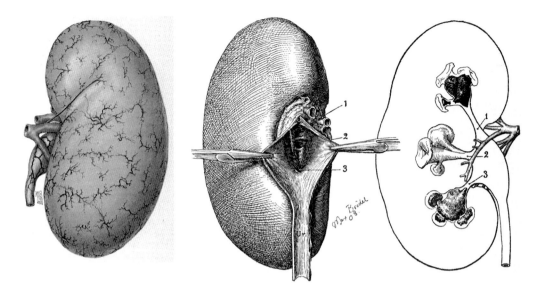

Max Brödel. *Left:* Fig. 179. The intrinsic blood vessels of the kidney and their significance in nephrotomy, 1901. Plate XXXIII (Figure 7A): A normal left kidney. *Right:* In Howard A. Kelly, *Diseases of the Kidneys, Ureters, and Bladder, with Special Reference to the Diseases of Women,* 1922. Figure 212: Kidneys with stones in upper and lower calices, with narrow necks. Note the lifelike appearance of the carbon dust illustration on the left, the clean lines of the textured pen-and-ink image in the middle, and the simplified drawing on the right. The latter shows little extraneous detail, and the kidney itself is suggested by a single contour line, yet none of the important details are lost in the process.

Historically, individually wood-carved crosshatches would be fragile, and having them attached on one side made the wood block sturdier. Unless one uses a beveled calligraphy pen, this technique is tedious and labor-intensive, but results in a classic and classy illustration. Almost as tedious is stippling, as used for the nasotracheal tube-securing strips of tape in Fig. 178—a "graying out" of the surface with a multitude of small dots. It is not a very difficult technique to master (if one has the patience and wrist stamina), and one that produces nuanced surface rendering.

The most commonly used method of texturing is cross-hatching, the placement of countless parallel lines to indicate gray tones. These lines can be straight, counting on the difference in overall tone to convey dark and light areas; or the lines can be curved, following the three-dimensional volume of the structure. For very large surfaces, the principle of cross-hatching can be used in small groups of five to ten short parallel lines, each group arranged in a random direction—a technique called basket hatching.

But if all that cross-hatching seems too labor-intensive, a neat short-cut is the answer: a few well-placed short, curvy lines that suggest a more extensive texture rendering. In the endotracheal tube example (Fig.

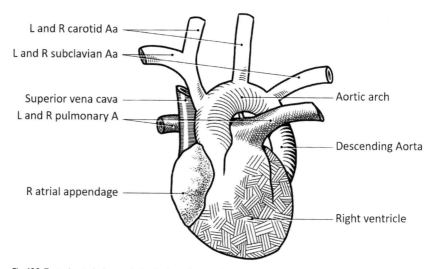

L and R carotid Aa

L and R subclavian Aa

Superior vena cava

L and R pulmonary A

R atrial appendage

Aortic arch

Descending Aorta

Right ventricle

Fig. 180: Texturing techniques, clockwise from: Descending aorta: "Woodcut" with variable line thickness. Right ventricle: Basket hatching, ideal for large surfaces. Atrial appendage: Stippling technique, which allows gradients of shading. Pulmonary artery: Cross-hatching. Superior vena cava: Hatching with straight parallel lines to give a uniform gray tone. Subclavian and carotid arteries: "Eyelashes," a shortcut to indicate volume with only a few hatching marks. Aortic arch: Hatching with curved parallel lines that add to the impression of volume by echoing the convexity of the structure.

176), the cartilaginous rings of the trachea appear three-dimensional simply by judiciously placed lines on the shady side of the structure (since the rings are convex and light is assumed to come from the top left, the lines are found on the right). These lines are colloquially known as *eyelashes*.[3]

Many clinicians may feel intimidated by the skills necessary to draw effectively. Medical illustrators are artists first, and it is very hard to compete with them. And yet, draw we do: most physicians use visual aids in their daily practice. The aim is not to create a masterpiece, but to make oneself understood, so much so that as Holly Quinton, a general practitioner who is also a graduate of the Glasgow School of Art, confesses, "some of [my] sketches stop 'mid drawing' as there is no need to continue. The image has served its purpose: to fill a small gap of knowledge or to reinforce a health education point."[4] Not only does it make it easier to communicate with patients, students, and peers but there is ample research evidence that it improves our own understanding of the concepts we are trying to explain.[5] And while we may not have the artistic eye of professional illustrators, we can all try to improve our skills. Giving volume to simple geometric shapes is not that difficult, and using simple tricks to enhance a drawing can even be fun. Of course, organs are not typically cubes or spheres, but

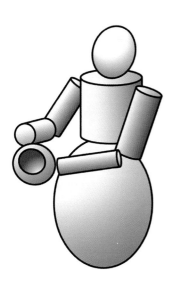

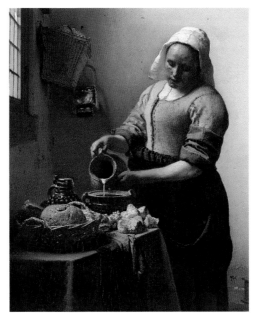

Fig. 181: When drawing complex structures or organs, it is easier to break them down into simple volumes, the better to sketch broad contours, shades, and shadows. Even a masterwork of classic art, like Johannes Vermeer's *Het Melkmeisje* (The milkmaid), can be reduced to spheres, ellipsoids, cylinders, cubes, and prisms.

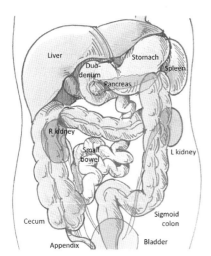

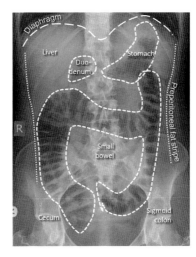

Fig. 182: Drawing detailed anatomy can be intimidating, but radiographs and other diagnostic images can help. For example, a simple abdominal X-ray shows the gas pattern in the stomach, duodenum, small bowel, and colon; the preperitoneal fat stripes and the diaphragm, which allows the medical professional/amateur illustrator to extrapolate the relative sizes and relationships of the solid and hollow organs.

the principles are the same, and organs and other complex structures can be deconstructed into basic volumes and shapes (Fig. 181). Our knowledge of anatomy and physiology (or any other discipline in our own specialty) are clearly assets. If we don't quite know how to draw the abdominal organs and their relationship to each other, for example, why not use a radiograph as a cheat sheet (Fig. 182)?

Physicians must be clear communicators, a trait they share with medical illustrators. Medical illustration is inextricably tied to science and medicine, and that collaboration is beneficial to both parties. From illustrators, we can learn an analytic approach to the dissemination of complex information—from the preliminary sketch and the level of detail to the clear narrative and the crisp images. We, too, can use visual communication to explain or teach, and to cut through the jargon and the language barriers. If we use drawings professionally, the same themes will show up repeatedly, and we will hone our skills, even if our range of illustrations remains narrow. With a little practice, cardiologists can develop their go-to sketch of a four-chamber heart, gastroenterologists can master a schematic GI tract, pathologists a cell with its organelles. The ultimate goal is to communicate, and as Mike Rohde observes in his books about Sketchnotes, there is little difference between a good drawing of a dog and a bad drawing of a dog—either way, it's still a dog.[6]

Notes

Introduction

1. Andreas Vesalius, Daniel H. Garrison, and Malcolm H. Hast, *The Fabric of the Human Body: An Annotated Translation of the 1543 and 1555 Editions of "De Humani Corporis Fabrica Libri Septem"* (Basel: S. Karger, 2014).

2. Francine M. Netter and Gary E. Friedlaender, "Frank H. Netter MD and a Brief History of Medical Illustration," *Clinical Orthopaedics and Related Research* 472, no. 3 (2014): 812–9, https://doi.org/10.1007/s11999-013-3459-8.

3. Berardo Di Matteo, Vittorio Tarabella, Giuseppe Filardo, Patrizia Tomba, Anna Vigano, and Maurillio Marcacci, "Nicolaes Tulp: The Overshadowed Subject in *The Anatomy Lesson of Dr. Nicolaes Tulp,*" *Clinical Orthopaedics and Related Research* 474, no. 3 (2016): 625–29, https://doi.org/10.1007/s11999-015-4686-y.

4. Lucas Boer, Anna B. Radziun, and Roelof-Jan Oostra, "Frederik Ruysch (1638–1731): Historical Perspective and Contemporary Analysis of His Teratological Legacy," *American Journal of Medical Genetics A* 173, no. 1 (2017): 16–41, https://doi.org/10.1002/ajmg.a.37663. Frank F. Ijpma and Thomas M. van Gulik, "Anatomy Lesson of Frederik Ruysch of 1670: A Tribute to Ruysch's Contributions to Lymphatic Anatomy," *World Journal of Surgery* 37, no. 8 (2013): 1996–2001, https://doi.org/10.1007/s00268 013 2013-x.

5. Marianne Berardi, *Science into Art: Rachel Ruysch's Early Development as a Still-life Painter* (Pittsburgh: Univ. of Pittsburgh, 1998), 595.

6. "Frederik Ruysch (1638–1731): Curator of Anatomical Specimens," *JAMA* 210, no. 3 (1969): 551, https://www.ncbi.nlm.nih.gov/pubmed/4899811.

7. Nora McGreevy, "For the First Time in Its 200-Year History, the Rijksmuseum Features Women Artists in 'Gallery of Honour,'" *Smithsonian Magazine,* Mar. 11, 2021, https://www.smithsonianmag.com/smart-news/rijksmuseum-will-display-work-women-artists-its-gallery-honour-first-time-180977209/.

8. Max Brodel, "Medical Illustration," *JAMA* 117, no. 9 (1941): 668–72, https://doi.org/10.1001/jama.1941.02820350008003. Reuben D. Johnson and Willow Sainsbury,

"The 'Combined Eye' of Surgeon and Artist: Evaluation of the Artists Who Illustrated for Cushing, Dandy and Cairns," *Journal of Clinical Neuroscience* 19, no. 1 (2012): 34–38, https://doi.org/10.1016/j.jocn.2011.03.042.

9. Melina Klepsch, Florian Schmitz, and Tina Seufert, "Development and Validation of Two Instruments Measuring Intrinsic, Extraneous, and Germane Cognitive Load," *Frontiers in Psychology* 8 (2017): 1997, https://doi.org/10.3389/fpsyg.2017.01997.

10. Constantine Mavroudis, Gary P. Lees, and Rachid Idriss, "Medical Illustration in the Era of Cardiac Surgery," *World Journal for Pediatric & Congenital Heart Surgery* 11, no. 2 (2020): 204–14, https://doi.org/10.1177/2150135119893671.

11. Kevin T. Liou, Paul George, Jay M. Baruch, and François I. Luks, "Clinical Sketches: Teaching Medical Illustration to Medical Students," *Medical Education* 48, no. 5 (2014): 525, https://doi.org/10.1111/medu.12450.

12. Christopher A. Stone, "Can a Picture Really Paint a Thousand Words?," *Aesthetic and Plastic Surgery* 24, no. 3 (2000): 185–91, https://doi.org/10.1007/s002660010030.

13. Nobuyuki Nakajima, Jun Wada, Tamotsu Miki, Jo Haraoka, and Nobuhiko Hata, "Surface Rendering-Based Virtual Intraventricular Endoscopy: Retrospective Feasibility Study and Comparison to Volume Rendering-Based Approach," Supplement, *Neuroimage* 37, S1 (2007): S89–99, https://doi.org/10.1016/j.neuroimage.2007.04.023.

14. Scott A. Collins, Jing Wu, and Harrison X. Bai, "Facial De-identification of Head CT Scans," *Radiology* 296, no. 1 (2020): 192617, https://doi.org/10.1148/radiol.2020192617.

15. François I. Luks, Scott Collins, Jimmy Xia, Shiliang A. Cao, and Matthew Rios, "Combination of Volume-Rendering 3D Surface Modeling and Medical Illustration to Capture the Living Fetus," *Prenatal Diagnosis* 41, no. 1 (2021): 79–88, https://doi.org/10.1002/pd.5844.

16. Alina Krasnoryadtseva, Nicola Dalbeth, and Keith J. Petrie, "The Effect of Different Styles of Medical Illustration on Information Comprehension, the Perception of Educational Material and Illness Beliefs," *Patient Education and Counseling* 103, no. 3 (2020): 556–62, https://doi.org/10.1016/j.pec.2019.09.026.

17. Mavroudis, Lees, and Idriss, "Medical Illustration in the Era of Cardiac Surgery."

18. Christoph Niemann, "You Are Fluent in This Language (and Don't Even Know It)," TED, https://www.ted.com/talks/christoph_niemann_you_are_fluent_in_this_language_and_don_t_even_know_it.

19. Holly Quinton, "Why I Use Drawing and Creative Processes during the GP Consultation," *British Journal of General Practice* 70, no. 700 (2020): 550, https://doi.org/10.3399/bjgp20X713273. Helene Cole, "Frank Netter, MD, 'Command Performance' in Medical Art," *JAMA* 255, no. 16 (1986): 2121–27, https://www.ncbi.nlm.nih.gov/pubmed/3514974. Julien Bogousslavsky and François Boller, "Jean-Martin Charcot and Art: Relationship of the 'Founder of Neurology' with Various Aspects of Art," *Progress in Brain Research* 203 (2013): 185–99, https://doi.org/10.1016/B978-0-444-62730-8.00007-4. Liou, George, Baruch, and Luks, "Clinical Sketches," 525.

20. Liou, George, Baruch, and Luks, "Clinical Sketches," 525. Sayra M. Cristancho, Susan J. Bidinosti, Lorelei A. Lingard, Richard J. Novick, Michael C. Ott, and Tom L. Forbes, "What's behind the Scenes? Exploring the Unspoken Dimensions of Complex and Challenging Surgical Situations," *Academic Medicine* 89, no. 11 (2014): 1540–47, https://doi.org/10.1097/ACM.0000000000000478.

21. Casey Lesser, "Why Med Schools Are Requiring Art Classes," https://www.artsy.net/article/artsy-editorial-med-schools-requiring-art-classes. John H. Kearsley, "Rembrandt, Michelangelo, and Stories of Healing," *Journal of Pain and Symptom Management* 42, no. 4 (2011): 783–87, https://doi.org/10.1016/j.jpainsymman.2011.05.004. Salvatore Mangione, Chayan Chakraborti, Giuseppe Staltari, Rebecca Harrison, Allan R. Tunkel, Kevin T. Liou, Elizabeth Cerceo, Megan Voeller, Wendy L. Bedwell, Keaton Fletcher, and Marc J. Kahn, "Medical Students' Exposure to the Humanities Correlates with Positive Personal Qualities and Reduced Burnout: A Multi-Institutional U.S. Survey," *Journal of General Internal Medicine* 33, no. 5 (2018): 628–34, https://doi.org/10.1007/s11606-017-4275-8.

22. Amy E. Herman, *Visual Intelligence: Sharpen Your Perception, Change Your Life* (New York: Eamon Dolan/Houghton Mifflin Harcourt, 2016).

1. The History of Medical Illustration

1. Harry McGurk and John MacDonald, "Hearing Lips and Seeing Voices," *Nature* 264, no. 5588 (1976): 746–48, https://doi.org/10.1038/264746a0.

2. Alina Krasnoryadtseva, Nicola Dalbeth, and Keith J. Petrie, "The Effect of Different Styles of Medical Illustration on Information Comprehension, the Perception of Educational Material and Illness Beliefs," *Patient Education and Counseling* 103, no. 3 (2020): 556–62, https://doi.org/10.1016/j.pec.2019.09.026.

3. Rachel Hajar, "Medical Illustration: Art in Medical Education," *Heart Views* 12, no. 2 (2011): 83–91, https://doi.org/10.4103/1995-705X.86023.

4. Kathleen Kuiper, "Venus of Willendorf," *Encyclopaedia Britannica* (Chicago: Encyclopaedia Britannica, Inc., 2018).

5. Francesco M. Galassi, Michael E. Habicht, and Frank J. Rühli, "Poliomyelitis in Ancient Egypt?," *Neurological Sciences* 38, no. 2 (2017): 375–75, https://doi.org/10.1007/s10072-016-2720-9.

6. David S. Kushner, John W. Verano, and Anne R. Titelbaum, "Trepanation Procedures/Outcomes: Comparison of Prehistoric Peru with Other Ancient, Medieval, and American Civil War Cranial Surgery," *World Neurosurgery* 114 (2018): 245–51, https://doi.org/10.1016/j.wneu.2018.03.143. Gregory Tsoucalas, Antonis A. Kousoulis, Theodoros Mariolis-Sapsakos, and Markos Sgantzos, "Trepanation Practices in Asclepieia: Systematizing a Neurosurgical Innovation," *World Neurosurgery* 103 (2017): 501–3, https://doi.org/10.1016/j.wneu.2017.04.022. Arthur S. Macnalty, "Vicary Lecture for 1945: The Renaissance and Its Influence on English Medicine Surgery and Public Health," *Annals of the Royal College of Surgeons of England* 1, no. 1 (1947): 8–30, https://www.ncbi.nlm.nih.gov/pubmed/19309813.

7. Kyeong-Seok Lee, "History of Chronic Subdural Hematoma," *Korean Journal of Neurotrauma* 11, no. 2 (2015): 27–34, https://doi.org/10.13004/kjnt.2015.11.2.27.

8. Susanna Collado-Vazquez and Jesus M. Carrillo, "Cranial Trepanation in the Egyptian," *Neurologia* 29, no. 7 (2014): 433–40, https://doi.org/10.1016/j.nrl.2011.05.012.

9. Macnalty, "The Renaissance and Its Influence," 8–30.

10. Norman M. Rich and Peter Rhee, "An Historical Tour of Vascular Injury Management: From Its Inception to the New Millennium," *Surgical Clinics of North America* 81, no. 6 (2001): 1199–215, https://doi.org/10.1016/s0039-6109(01)80005-0.

11. Macnalty, "The Renaissance and Its Influence," 8–30.

12. Evelyne Berriot-Salvadore, "'A Recollection': The Arrangement of Ambroise Paré's *Oeuvres*," *Etudes Françaises* 38, no. 3 (2002): 81–92, https://www.ncbi.nlmnih. gov/pubmed/18038488.

13. Chiara Benati, "Physical Impairment in the First Surgical Handbooks Printed in Germany," in *Fifteenth-Century Studies 35,* ed. M. Z. Heintzelman, B. I. Gusick, and M. W. Walsh (Rochester: Boydell & Brewer, 2010), 12–22.

14. Macnalty, "The Renaissance and Its Influence," 8–30.

15. H. Gaston Hall, "Molière Satirist of Seventeenth-Century French Medicine: Fact and Fantasy," *Proceedings of the Royal Society of Medicine* 70, no. 6 (1977): 425–31, https://doi.org/10.1177/003591577707000617.

16. John Harington, *The School of Salernum* (New York: Paul B. Hoeber, 1920). Johannes H. Baas, *Outlines of the History of Medicine and the Medical Profession* (New York: J. H. Vail, 1889).

17. Roberto Bolli, "William Harvey and the Discovery of the Circulation of the Blood," *Circulation Research* 124, no. 8 (2019): 1300–1302, https://doi.org/10.1161/ circresaha.119.314976.

18. Patrice Le Floch-Prigent, "Un Mannequin Anatomique en Ivoire" [An ivory visceral anatomic mannequin], *Acta Anatomica* 136, no. 2 (1989): 142–45, https:// www.ncbi.nlm.nih.gov/pubmed/2683554.

19. Andrea A. Conti and Ferdinando Paternostro, "Anatomical Study in the Western World before the Middle Ages: Historical Evidence," *Acta Biomedica* 90, no. 4 (2019): 523–25, https://doi.org/10.23750/abm.v90i4.8738. Vivian Nutton, "Portraits of Science: Logic, Learning, and Experimental Medicine," *Science* 295, no. 5556 (2002): 800–801, https://doi.org/10.1126/science.1066244.

20. Heinrich von Staden, "The Discovery of the Body: Human Dissection and Its Cultural Contexts in Ancient Greece," *Yale Journal of Biology and Medicine* 65, no. 3 (1992): 223–41, https://www.ncbi.nlm.nih.gov/pubmed/1285450.

21. Charles Daremberg, *Les Aphorismes d'Hippocrate* [Aphorisms by Hippocrates] (Paris: A l'enseigne du pot cassé, 1945).

22. Charles M. Goss and Elizabeth G. Chodkowski, "Whether Blood Is Contained in the Arteries of the Living Animal by Galen of Pergamon: A Translation," *Anatomical Record* 213, no. 1 (1985): 1–6, https://doi.org/10.1002/ar.1092130102.

23. Malak A. Alghamdi, Janine M. Ziermann, and Rui Diogo, "An Untold Story: The Important Contributions of Muslim Scholars for the Understanding of Human Anatomy," *Anatomical Record* 300, no. 6 (2017), https://doi.org/10.1002/ar.23523. M. Akmal, Mohd Zulkifle, and Abdul H. Ansari, "Ibn Nafis—A Forgotten Genius in the Discovery of Pulmonary Blood Circulation," *Heart Views* 11, no. 1 (2010): 26–30, https://www.ncbi.nlm.nih.gov/pubmed/21042463. Izet Masic, "On Occasion of 800th Anniversary of Birth of Ibn al-Nafis—Discoverer of Cardiac and Pulmonary Circulation," *Medicinski Arhiv* 64, no. 5 (2010): 309–13, https://doi.org/10.5455/ medarh.2010.64.

24. Arman Zargaran, "Avicenna or Ibn Nafis; Who Did Mention to the Role of Coronary Arteries in Blood Supply of the Heart?," *International Journal of Cardiology* 247 (2017): 47, https://doi.org/10.1016/j.ijcard.2017.06.093.

25. Akmal, Zulkifle, and Ansari, "Ibn Nafis," 26–30. Masic, "On Occasion of 800th Anniversary of Birth of Ibn al-Nafis."

26. Hasan F. Batirel, "Early Islamic Physicians and Thorax," *Annals of Thoracic Surgery* 67, no. 2 (1999): 578–80, https://doi.org/10.1016/s0003-4975(98)01295-8.

27. von Staden, "The Discovery of the Body," 223–41.

28. Salih M. Akkin and Gulten Dinc, "A Glimpse into the Process of Gaining Permission for the Educational Dissection of Human Cadavers in the Ottoman Empire," *Clinical Anatomy* 27, no. 7 (2014): 964–71, https://doi.org/10.1002/ca.22421.

29. Mohammadali M. Shoja and R. Shane Tubbs, "The History of Anatomy in Persia," *Journal of Anatomy* 210, no. 4 (2007): 359–78, https://doi.org/10.1111/j.1469-7580.2007.00711.x.

30. von Staden, "The Discovery of the Body," 223–41.

31. Spyros Retsas, "Galen's 'Errors,'" *Lancet* 376, no. 9742 (2010): 686, https://doi.org/10.1016/S0140-6736(10)61337-2. Gül A. Russell, "Vesalius and the Emergence of Veridical Representation in Renaissance Anatomy," *Progress in Brain Research* 203 (2013): 3–32, https://doi.org/10.1016/B978-0-444-62730-8.00001-3.

32. Katherine Park, *Secrets of Women: Gender, Generation, and the Origins of Human Dissection* (Cambridge, MA: MIT Press, 2006).

33. André Parent, "Berengario da Carpi and the Renaissance of Brain Anatomy," *Frontiers in Neuroanatomy* 13 (2019): 1–14, https://doi.org/10.3389/fnana.2019.00011.

34. Francisco Guerra, "The Identity of the Artists Involved in Vesalius's *Fabrica* 1543," *Medical History* 13, no. 1 (1969): 37–50, https://doi.org/10.1017/S0025727300013934.

35. Omar Habbal, "The Science of Anatomy: A Historical Timeline," *Sultan Qaboos University Medical Journal* 17, no. 1 (2017): e18–e22, https://doi.org/10.18295/squmj.2016.17.01.004.

36. Guerra, "Identity of the Artists Involved," 37–50.

37. Linda Wilson-Pauwels, "Jan Wandelaar, Bernard Siegfried Albinus and an Indian Rhinoceros Named Clara Set High Standards as the Process of Anatomical Illustration Entered a New Phase of Precision, Artistic Beauty, and Marketing in the 18th Century," *Journal of Biocommunication* 35, n0.1 (2009): E10–E17.

38. Wilson-Pauwels, "Jan Wandelaar, Bernard Siegfried Albinus and an Indian Rhinoceros Named Clara."

39. James Elkins, "Two Conceptions of the Human Form: Bernard Siegfried Albinus and Andreas Vesalius," *Artibus et Historiae* 7, no. 14 (1986): 91–106, https://doi.org/10.2307/1483226.

40. Domenico B. Meli, *Visualizing Disease: The Art and History of Pathological Illustrations* (Chicago: University of Chicago Press, 2018).

41. Raymond Lifchez, "Jean-Galbert Salvage and His *Anatomie du gladiateur combattant:* Art and Patronage in Post-Revolutionary France," *Metropolitan Museum Journal* 44 (2009): 163–84, www.jstor.org/stable/25699111.

42. Jonathan R. Hiatt and Nathan Hiatt, "The Forgotten First Career of Doctor Henry Van Dyke Carter," *Journal of the American College of Surgeons* 181, no. 5 (1995): 464–66, https://www.ncbi.nlm.nih.gov/pubmed/7582216.

43. Wendy K. Moore, *The Knife Man: The Extraordinary Life and Times of John Hunter, Father of Modern Surgery* (New York: Broadway Books, 2005).

44. Jean-Baptiste M. Bourgery, Nicolas H. Jacob, Jean-Marie L. Minor, and Henri Sick, *Atlas d'Anatomie Humaine et de Chirurgie* [Atlas of human anatomy and surgery] (Cologne: Taschen, 2012), introduction.

45. Reinhard Hildebrand, "Anatomie und Revolution des Menschenbildes" [Anatomy and revolution of the human image], *Sudhoffs Archiv* 76, no. 1 (1992): 1–27.

46. Max Brodel. "Medical Illustration," *JAMA* 117, no. 9 (1941): 668–72, https://doi.org/10.1001/jama.1941.02820350008003. Reuben D. Johnson and Willow Sainsbury, "The 'Combined Eye' of Surgeon and Artist: Evaluation of the Artists Who Illustrated for Cushing, Dandy and Cairns," *Journal of Clinical Neuroscience* 19, no. 1 (2012):

34–38, https://doi.org/10.1016/j.jocn.2011.03.042. Ranice W. Crosby and John Cody, *Max Brödel: The Man Who Put Art into Medicine* (New York: Springer, 2011).

47. Brodel, "Medical Illustration."

2. The Accidental Medical Illustrator

1. Carlos A. Rodriguez, Carolina Isaza, and Harry Pachajoa, "Achondroplasia among Ancient Populations of Mesoamerica and South America: Iconographic and Archaeological Evidence," *Colombia Médica* 43, no. 2 (2012): 212–15, https://www.ncbi.nlm.nih.gov/pubmed/24893194. James C. Harris, "Portrait of Francisco Lezcano—the 'Nino de Vallecas,'" *Archives of General Psychiatry* 68, no. 3 (2011): 229, https://doi.org/10.1001/archgenpsychiatry.2011.13. John M Starbuck, "On the Antiquity of Trisomy 21: Moving towards a Quantitative Diagnosis of Down Syndrome in Historic Material Culture," *Journal of Contemporary Anthropology* 2, no. 1 (2011): 18–44. Andrew S. Levitas and Cheryl S. Reid, "An Angel with Down Syndrome in a Sixteenth-Century Flemish Nativity Painting," *American Journal of Medical Genetics A* 116A, no. 4 (2003): 399–405, https://doi.org/10.1002/ajmg.a.10043.

2. Frank L. Meshberger, "An Interpretation of Michelangelo's Creation of Adam Based on Neuroanatomy," *JAMA* 264, no. 14 (1990): 1837–41, https://www.ncbi.nlm.nih.gov/pubmed/2205727. Ian Suk and Rafael J. Tamargo, "Concealed Neuroanatomy in Michelangelo's *Separation of Light from Darkness* in the Sistine Chapel," *Neurosurgery* 66, no. 5 (2010): 851–61, https://doi.org/10.1227/01.NEU.0000368101.34523.E1.

3. Suk and Tamargo, "Concealed Neuroanatomy."

4. Victoria Avery and Paul Joannides, *A Michelangelo Discovery: The Rothschild Bronzes and the Case for Their Proposed Attribution* (Oxford: Fitzwilliam Museum, 2015).

5. Sayra M. Cristancho, Susan J. Bidinosti, Lorelei A. Lingard, Richard J. Novick, Michael C. Ott, and Tom L. Forbes, "What's behind the Scenes? Exploring the Unspoken Dimensions of Complex and Challenging Surgical Situations," *Academic Medicine* 89, no. 11 (2014): 1540–7, https://doi.org/10.1097/ACM.0000000000000478. Amit Om and Anjali Om, "Integrating the Integumentary System with the Arts: A Review of Dermatologic Findings in Artwork," *Journal of Clinical Aesthetic Dermatology* 11, no. 9 (2018): 21–27, https://www.ncbi.nlm.nih.gov/pubmed/30319727. Christine Digrazia, "Yale's Life-or-Death Course in Art Criticism," *New York Times,* National ed., May 19, 2002, 14.

6. Casey Lesser, "Why Med Schools Are Requiring Art Classes," https://www.artsy.net/article/artsy-editorial-med-schools-requiring-art-classes. John H. Kearsley, "Rembrandt, Michelangelo, and Stories of Healing," *Journal of Pain and Symptom Management* 42, no. 5 (2011): 783–87, https://doi.org/10.1016/j.jpainsymman.2011.05.004.

7. Salvatore Mangione, Chayan Chakraborti, Giuseppe Staltari, Rebecca Harrison, Allan R. Tunkel, Kevin T. Liou, Elizabeth Cerceo, Megan Voeller, Wendy L. Bedwell, Keaton Fletcher, and Marc J. Kahn, "Medical Students' Exposure to the Humanities Correlates with Positive Personal Qualities and Reduced Burnout: A Multi-Institutional U.S. Survey," *Journal of General Internal Medicine* 33, no. 5 (2018): 628–34, https://doi.org/10.1007/s11606-017-4275-8.

8. Stefan Riedel, "Edward Jenner and the History of Smallpox and Vaccination," *Baylor University Medical Center Proceedings* 18, no. 1 (2005): 21–25, https://doi.org/10.1080/08998280.2005.11928028.

9. World Health Assembly, *Declaration of Global Eradication of Smallpox* (Geneva: World Health Organization, 1980).

10. Donatella Lippi, John P. D'Elios, and Saverio Caini, "Smallpox in the Medici Family, Florence, 1519–1737: A Historical Cohort Study," *Clinical Microbiology and Infection* 21, no. 8 (2015): PE57–PE58, https://doi.org/10.1016/j.cmi.2015.01.021.

11. Jesse D. Bloom, Yujia A. Chan, Ralph S. Baric, et al., "Investigate the Origins of COVID-19," *Science* 372, no. 6543 (2021): 694, https://doi.org/10.1126/science.abj0016.

12. Jean-Jacques Battin, "Le Feu Saint-Antoine ou Ergotisme Gangréneux et son Iconographie Médiévale" [Antony's fire (gangrenous ergotism) and medieval iconography], *Bulletin de l'Académie Nationale de Médecine* 193, no. 8 (2009): 1925–36, https://www.ncbi.nlm.nih.gov/pubmed/20669555.

13. John Goldie, "The Implications of Brain Lateralisation for Modern General Practice," *The British Journal of General Practice: The Journal of the Royal College of General Practitioners* 66, no. 642 (2016): 44–45, https://doi.org/10.3399/bjgp16X683341. Sean Hughes and Christopher Gardner-Thorpe, "Charles Bell (1774–1842) and Natural Theology," *Journal of Medical Biography* 28, no. 2 (2020): 75–82, https://doi.org/10.1177/0967772018790736.

14. Ronnie Henry, "Etymologia: Poliomyelitis," *Emerging Infectious Diseases* 25, no. 8 (2019): 1611, https://doi.org/10.3201/eid2508.ET2508.

15. Paul Richer and Robern B. Hale, *Artistic Anatomy* (New York: Watson-Guptill Publications, 1986).

16. Arthur W. Boylston, "The Myth of the Milkmaid," *New England Journal of Medicine* 378, no. 5 (2018): 414–15, https://doi.org/10.1056/NEJMp1715349.

17. Robert S. Morton, "Syphilis in Art: An Entertainment in Four Parts," pt 4, *Genitourinary Medicine* 66, no. 4 (1990): 280–94, https://doi.org/10.1136/sti.66.4.280.

18. Robert S. Morton, "Syphilis in Art: An Entertainment in Four Parts," pt 1, *Genitourinary Medicine* 66, no. 1 (1990): 33–40, https://doi.org/10.1136/sti.66.1.33.

19. Robert S. Morton, "Syphilis in Art: An Entertainment in Four Parts," pt 3, *Genitourinary Medicine* 66, no. 3 (1990): 208–21, https://doi.org/10.1136/sti.66.3.208.

20. Frank F. Ijpma and Thomas M. van Gulik, "Bidloo's and de Lairesse's Early Illustrations of the Anatomy of the Arm (1690): A Successful Collaboration between a Prominent Physician and a Talented Artist," *The Journal of Hand Surgery,* 38, no. 1 (2013): 97–99, https://doi.org/10.1177/1753193412454396. Jan C. Molenaar, "Anatomie als Schouwspel. Uit de Bibliotheek van de Vereniging Nederlands Tijdschrift voor Geneeskunde. Govard Bidloo: Ontleding des Menschelijken Lichaams, 1689; en William Cowper: The Anatomy of Humane Bodies," 1698 [Anatomy as theatre]. From the library of the Society of the Dutch Journal of Medicine. Govard Bidloo, *Dissection of the Human Body,* 1689; and William Cowper, *The Anatomy of Humane Bodies,* 1698. *Nederlands tijdschrift voor geneeskunde* 148, no. 52 (2004): 2594–602.

21. Morton, "Syphilis in Art," pt 3. Horton A. Johnson, "Gerard de Lairesse: Genius among the Treponemes," *Journal of the Royal Society of Medicine* 97, no. 6 (2004): 301–3, https://doi.org/10.1258/jrsm.97.6.301.

22. Stephen McWilliams, *Fiction and Physicians: Medicine Through the Eyes of Writers* (Dublin: Liffey Press, 2012).

23. Brian Livesley, *The Dying Keats: A Case for Euthanasia?* (Leicester: Troubador Publishing Limited, 2009).

24. Brian Livesley, "'Little Keats' and His Congenital Diseases," *Bulletin of the Royal College of Surgeons of England* 94, no. 4 (2012): 1–7, https://doi.org/10.1308/147363512X13189526440519.

25. Om and Om, "Integrating the Integumentary System with the Arts," 21–27.

26. Mark Tan, Samantha Goh, and Hutan Ashrafian, "Michelangelo's John the Baptist and Thalassemia," *Annals of Hematology* 92, no. 9 (2013): 1293–94, https://doi.org/10.1007/s00277-013-1710-8.

27. Gerald D. Hart, "The Habsburg Jaw," *Canadian Medical Association Journal* 104, no. 7 (1971): 601–3, https://www.ncbi.nlm.nih.gov/pubmed/4927696.

28. Gerald P. Hodge, "A Medical History of the Spanish Habsburgs: As Traced in Portraits," *JAMA* 238, no. 11 (1977): 1169–74, https://doi.org/10.1001/jama.1977.03280120061018. Gonzalo Álvarez and Francisco C. Ceballos, "Royal Inbreeding and the Extinction of Lineages of the Habsburg Dynasty," *Human Heredity* 80, no. 2 (2015): 62–68, https://doi.org/10.1159/000440765.

29. McWilliams, *Fiction and Physicians*.

30. Zachary S. Peacock, Katherine P. Klein, John B. Mulliken, and Leonard B. Kaban, "The Habsburg Jaw Re-examined," *American Journal of Medical Genetics A* 164a, no. 9 (2014): 2263–69, https://doi.org/10.1002/ajmg.a.36639.

31. Rashid M. Rashid and Len E. White, "A Hairy Development in Hypertrichosis: A Brief Review of Ambras Syndrome," *Dermatology Online Journal* 13, no. 3 (2007): 8, https://www.ncbi.nlm.nih.gov/pubmed/18328202.

32. Camille Zabka, *Les Monstres et l'Humain—si Proc hes, si Lointains* [Monsters and the human: So close, so far] (Paris: J'ai lu, 2016).

33. Harry Angelman, "'Puppet' Children: A Report on Three Cases," *Developmental Medicine & Child Neurology* 7, no. 6 (1965): 681–88, https://doi.org/10.1111/j.1469-8749.1965.tb07844.x.

34. Nenad Bukvic and John W. Elling, "Genetics in the Art and Art in Genetics," *Gene* 555, no. 1 (2015): 14–22, https://doi.org/10.1016/j.gene.2014.07.073.

35. Suzanne B. Cassidy and Stuart Schwartz, "Prader-Willi and Angelman Syndromes: Disorders of Genomic Imprinting," *Medicine* 77, no. 2 (1998), https://journals.lww.com/md-journal/Fulltext/1998/03000/Prader_Willi_and_Angelman_Syndromes__Disorders_of.5.aspx.

36. Carlos M. Oranges, Mirjam Christ-Crain, and Dirk J. Schaefer, "'La Monstrua Desnuda': An Artistic Textbook Representation of Prader-Willi Syndrome in a Painting of Juan Carreño de Miranda (1680)," *Journal of Endocrinological Investigation* 40, no. 6 (2017): 691–92, https://doi.org/10.1007/s40618-017-0639-5. Merlin G. Butler, Phillip D. K. Lee and Barbara Y. Whitman, *Management of Prader-Willi Syndrome* (New York: Springer, 2006).

37. Bruce D. Gelb, Guo-Ping Shi, Harold A. Chapman, and Robert J. Desnick, "Pycnodysostosis, a Lysosomal Disease Caused by Cathepsin K Deficiency," *Science* 273, no. 5279 (1996): 1236–38, https://doi.org/10.1126/science.273.5279.1236.

38. Ad A. Kaptein, Pim B. van der Meer, Barend W. Florijn, Alexander D. Hilt, Michael Murray, and Martin J. Schalij, "Heart in Art: Cardiovascular Diseases in Novels, Films, and Paintings," *Philosophy, Ethics, and Humanities in Medicine* 15, no. 1 (2020): 1–10, https://doi.org/10.1186/s13010-020-0086-3.

39. W. H. de Haas, "Dick Ket, een Schilder en zijn Ziekte" [Dick Ket, a painter and his illness], *Nederlands Tijdschrift voor Geneeskunde* 128, no. 51 (1984): 2423–25.

40. Alfred Blalock and Helen B. Taussig, "The Surgical Treatment of Malformations of the Heart in Which There Is Pulmonary Stenosis or Pulmonary Atresia," *JAMA* 251, no. 16 (1984): 2123–38, https://doi.org/10.1001/jama.251.16.2123.

41. Valmantas Budrys, "Frida Kahlo's Neurological Deficits and Her Art," *Progress in Brain Research* 203 (2013): 241–54, https://doi.org/10.1016/B978-0-444-62730-8.00010-4.

42. Julian D. A. Wiseman, "What Malformation Did El Greco Paint?," Mar. 2020, http://www.jdawiseman.com/papers/el-greco/el-greco-dysmorphology.html.

43. Patrick Trevor-Roper, *The World through Blunted Sight: An Inquiry into the Influence of Defective Vision on Art and Character* (London: Profile, 2012).

44. Przemyslaw Prusinkiewicz and Enrico Coen, "Passing the El Greco Test," *Human Frontier Science Program Journal* 1, no. 3 (2007): 152–55, https://doi.org/10.2976/1.2776103.

45. Phillip Barcio, *The Evolution of Style in Piet Mondrian Artwork* (London: IdeelArt, 2016).

46. Michael F. Marmor, "Ophthalmology and Art: Simulation of Monet's Cataracts and Degas' Retinal Disease," *Archives of Ophthalmology* 124, no. 12 (2006): 1764–69, https://doi.org/10.1001/archopht.124.12.1764.

47. Marmor, "Ophthalmology and Art."

48. Anna Gruener, "The Effect of Cataracts and Cataract Surgery on Claude Monet," *British Journal of General Practice* 65, no. 634 (2015): 254–55, https://doi.org/10.3399/bjgp15X684949.

49. Lynn Eaton, "Former BMJ Artist Demonstrates the Effect of Cataract," *British Medical Journal* 334, no. 7586 (2007): 177, https://doi.org/10.1136/bmj.39104.432685.AB.

50. Kalyan B. Bhattacharyya and Saurabh Rai, "The Neuropsychiatric Ailment of Vincent van Gogh," *Annals of the Indian Academy of Neurology* 18, no. 1 (2015): 6–9, https://doi.org/10.4103/0972-2327.145286. Gabriele Bronzetti, "Il giallo digitale di Van Gogh e Pascoli" [Vincent van Gogh and Giovanni Pascoli, foiled by the foxglove], *Recenti Progressi in Medicina* 110, no. 5 (2019): 259–62, https://doi.org/10.1701/3163.31450.

51. Philippe Lanthony, "La Xanthopsie de Van Gogh" [Van Gogh's xanthopsia], *Bulletin de la Société Ophtalmologique Française* 89, no. 10 (1989): 1133–34, https://www.ncbi.nlm.nih.gov/pubmed/2695267.

52. Thomas C. Lee, "Van Gogh's Vision: Digitalis Intoxication?," *JAMA* 245, no. 7 (1981): 727–29, https://www.ncbi.nlm.nih.gov/pubmed/7007674.

53. Lee, "Van Gogh's Vision."

54. Wilfred N. Arnold and Loretta S. Loftus, "Xanthopsia and van Gogh's Yellow Palette," pt 5, *Eye* 5 (1991): 503–10, https://doi.org/10.1038/eye.1991.93.

55. Helene Cole, "Frank Netter, MD: 'Command Performance' in Medical Art," *JAMA* 255, no. 16 (1986): 2121–27, https://www.ncbi.nlm.nih.gov/pubmed/3514974.

56. Anna Gruener, "Munch's Visions from within the Eye," *British Journal of General Practice* 64, no. 618 (2014): 36–37, https://doi.org/10.3399/bjgp14X676492.

57. Geoffrey D. Schott, "The Sick Durer—A Renaissance Prototype Pain Map," *British Medical Journal* 329, no. 7480 (2004): 1492, https://doi.org/10.1136/bmj.329.7480.1492.

58. Victor A. McKusick, "Brödel's Ulnar Palsy: With Unpublished Brödel Sketches," *Bulletin of the History of Medicine* 23, no. 5 (1949): 469–79, www.jstor.org/stable/44442273.

59. Ugo F. Tesler, "The History of Art versus the Art of Surgery" *Texas Heart Institute Journal* 39, no. 6 (2012): 825–30, https://www.ncbi.nlm.nih.gov/pubmed/23304023.

60. Harold Ellis, *Operations That Made History* (Cambridge: Cambridge Univ. Press, 2009).

61. Kevin P. Lee, "Caroline Hampton Halsted and the Origin of Surgical Gloves," *Journal of Medical Biography* 28, no. 1 (2020): 64–66, https://doi.org/10.1177/0967772019869167.

62. Ira M. Rutkow, "The Surgeon's Glove," *Archives of Surgery* 134, no. 2 (1999): 223, https://doi.org/10.1001/archsurg.134.2.223.

63. Ellis, *Operations That Made History*. Jan Mikulicz, "Das Operieren in sterilisierten Zwirnhandschuhen und mit Augenbinde" [Operating with sterilized cloth gloves and eye protection], *Zentralblatt für Chirurgie* 24, no. 26 (1897): 713–17.

64. Colin Martin, "Cutting-Edge Art in the Operating Theatre," *Lancet* 363, no. 9411 (2004): 828, https://doi.org/10.1016/S0140-6736(04)15703-6.

3. The Shady Side of Medical Illustration

1. Peter J. Gartner, *Musée d'Orsay* (Potsdam: H. F. Ullman, 2001).

2. Pierre Cabanne, *"Le Scandale dans l'Art"* [Scandal in art] (Paris: La Différence, 2007).

3. Jonathan Jones, "Madame XXX," *Guardian,* Feb. 1, 2006, https://www.theguardian.com/culture/2006/feb/01/3.

4. Séverine Laborie, *Le Radeau de la* Méduse [The raft of the *Medusa*], https://www.louvre.fr/oeuvre-notices/le-radeau-de-la-meduse.

5. Paul Koudounaris, "Théodore Géricault's Morgue-Based Preparatory Paintings for 'Raft of the *Medusa,'*" *Morbid Anatomy,* Feb. 19, 2012, http://morbidanatomy.blogspot.com/2012/02/theodore-gericaults-morgue-based.html.

6. Heinrich von Staden, "The Discovery of the Body: Human Dissection and Its Cultural Contexts in Ancient Greece," *Yale Journal of Biology and Medicine* 65, no. 3 (1992): 223–41, https://www.ncbi.nlm.nih.gov/pubmed/1285450. Malak A. Alghamdi, Janine M. Ziermann, and Rui Diogo, "An Untold Story: The Important Contributions of Muslim Scholars for the Understanding of Human Anatomy," *Anatomical Record* 300, no. 6 (2017): 986–1008, https://doi.org/10.1002/ar.23523. Salih M. Akkin and Gulten Dinc, "A Glimpse into the Process of Gaining Permission for the Educational Dissection of Human Cadavers in the Ottoman Empire," *Clinical Anatomy* 27, no. 7 (2014): 964–71, https://doi.org/10.1002/ca.22421. Mohammadali M. Shoja and R. Shane Tubbs, "The History of Anatomy in Persia," *Journal of Anatomy* 210, no. 4 (2007): 359–78, https://doi.org/10.1111/j.1469-7580.2007.00711.x.

7. Katharine Park, *Secrets of Women: Gender, Generation, and the Origins of Human Dissection* (Cambridge, MA: MIT Press, 2006).

8. Bradford A. Bouley, *Pious Postmortems: Anatomy, Sanctity, and the Catholic Church in Early Modern Europe* (Philadelphia: Univ. of Pennsylvania Press, Inc., 2017).

9. Bouley, *Pious Postmortems*.

10. Park, *Secrets of Women*.

11. William Schupbach, "The Paradox of Rembrandt's 'Anatomy of Dr. Tulp,'" *Medical History* Supplement 2 (1982): 1–110, https://www.ncbi.nlm.nih.gov/pmc/articles/PMC2557395/.

12. Denis Dooley, "A Dissection of Anatomy," *Annals of the Royal College of Surgeons of England* 53, no. 1 (1973): 13–26, https://pubmed.ncbi.nlm.nih.gov/4579390.

13. Harold Ellis, "The Company of Barbers and Surgeons," *Journal of the Royal Society of Medicine* 94, no. 10 (2001): 548–49, https://www.ncbi.nlm.nih.gov/pmc/articles/PMC1282221/. Arthur S. Macnalty, "Vicary Lecture for 1945: The Renaissance and Its Influence on English Medicine Surgery and Public Health," *Annals of the Royal College of Surgeons of England* 1, no. 1 (1947): 8–30, https://www.ncbi.nlm.nih.gov/pubmed/19309813.

14. Wendy Moore, *The Knife Man: The Extraordinary Life and Times of John Hunter, Father of Modern Surgery* (New York: Broadway Books, 2005).

15. Kurt Kohlstedt, "Grave Guns & Coffin Torpedoes: Vintage Defenses Aimed to Foil Grave Robbers," https://99percentinvisible.org/article/grave-guns-coffin-torpedoes-vintage-defenses-aimed-foil-grave-robbers/.

16. Moore, *The Knife Man.*

17. Neil H. McAlister, "John Hunter and the Irish Giant," *Canadian Medical Association Journal* 111, no. 3 (1974): 256–77, https://www.ncbi.nlm.nih.gov/pubmed/4604654.

18. Mary B. Emmerichs, "Getting Away with Murder? Homicide and the Coroners in Nineteenth-Century London," *Social Science History* 25, no. 1 (2001): 93–100, https://doi.org/10.1215/01455532-25-1-93.

19. Dooley, "A Dissection of Anatomy."

20. Eli Y. Adashi, Leroy B. Walters, and Jerry A. Menikoff, "The Belmont Report at 40: Reckoning with Time," *American Journal of Public Health* 108, no. 10 (2018): 1345–48, https://doi.org/10.2105/ajph.2018.304580.

21. Richard S. Panush, "Nazi Origins of an Anatomy Text: The Pernkopf Atlas," *JAMA* 276, no. 20 (1996): 1633–34; author reply 1634, https://doi.org/10.1001/jama.1996.03540200019011. Howard A. Israel and William E. Seidelman, "Nazi Origins of an Anatomy Text: The Pernkopf Atlas," *JAMA* 276, no. 20 (1996): 1633 (Letter to the Editor), https://doi.org/10.1001/jama.276.20.1633b.

22. Andrew Yee, Ema Zubovic, Jennifer Yu, et al., "Ethical Considerations in the Use of Pernkopf's Atlas of Anatomy: A Surgical Case Study" *Surgery* 165, no. 5 (2019): 860–67, https://doi.org/10.1016/j.surg.2018.07.025.

23. Claude Vanderpooten, "Alexis Carrel: La Mystification . . ." [Alexis Carrell: The mystification . . .], *Histoire des Sciences Médicales* 30, no. 2 (1996): 155–61.

24. Chris Hubbard, "Eduard Pernkopf's Atlas of Topographical and Applied Human Anatomy: The Continuing Ethical Controversy," *Anatomical Record* 265, no. 5 (2001): 207–11, https://doi.org/10.1002/ar.1157.

25. Sabine Hildebrandt, "How the Pernkopf Controversy Facilitated a Historical and Ethical Analysis of the Anatomical Sciences in Austria and Germany: A Recommendation for the Continued Use of the Pernkopf Atlas," *Clinical Anatomy* 19, no. 2 (2006): 91–100, https://doi.org/10.1002/ca.20272.

26. Israel and Seidelman, "Nazi Origins of an Anatomy Text." Nicholas Wade, "Doctors Question Use of Nazi's Medical Atlas," *New York Times,* Nov. 26, 1996. Yee et al., "Ethical Considerations."

27. Yee et al., "Ethical Considerations."

28. Hildebrandt, "How the Pernkopf Controversy Facilitated a Historical and Ethical Analysis."

29. Herwig Czech and Erich Brenner, "Nazi Victims on the Dissection Table—The Anatomical Institute in Innsbruck," *Annals of Anatomy* 226 (2019): 84–95, https://doi.org/10.1016/j.aanat.2019.03.007.

30. Yee et al., "Ethical Considerations."

31. D. Gareth Jones, "Anatomy and Ethics: An Exploration of Some Ethical Dimensions of Contemporary Anatomy," *Clinical Anatomy* 11, no. 2 (1998): 100–105, https://doi.org/10.1002/(sici)1098-2353(1998)11:2<100::aid-ca6>3.0.co;2-y.

32. World Medical Association, "World Medical Association Declaration of Helsinki: Ethical Principles for Medical Research Involving Human Subjects," *JAMA* 310, no. 20 (2013): 2191–94, https://doi.org/10.1001/jama.2013.281053.

33. Adashi, Walters, and Menikoff, "The Belmont Report at 40."

34. Panush, "Nazi Origins of an Anatomy Text."

35. Garrett Riggs, "What Should We Do about Eduard Pernkopf's Atlas?," *Academic Medicine* 73, no. 4 (1998): 380–86, https://doi.org/10.1097/00001888-199804000-00010.

36. Hildebrandt, "How the Pernkopf Controversy Facilitated a Historical and Ethical Analysis."

37. Gabrielle Beaumont, "Great Balls Afire," in *L.A. Law,* season 6, episode 15, ed. Steven Bochco and Terry L. Fisher (Los Angeles: NBC, 1992), 47 minutes.

38. Yee et al. "Ethical Considerations."

39. Adam K. Raymond, "The Push to Not Name Mass Shooters Is Catching On," *New York Magazine,* May 9, 2019.

40. Yee et al., "Ethical Considerations."

41. Michel C. Atlas, "Ethics and Access to Teaching Materials in the Medical Library: The Case of the Pernkopf Atlas," *Bulletin of the Medical Library Association* 89, no. 1 (2001): 51–88, https://www.ncbi.nlm.nih.gov/pubmed/11209801.

42. Hubbard, *Eduard Pernkopf's Atlas.*

43. Panush, "Nazi Origins of an Anatomy Text."

44. Hildebrandt, "How the Pernkopf Controversy Facilitated a Historical and Ethical Analysis."

45. Hildebrandt, "How the Pernkopf Controversy Facilitated a Historical and Ethical Analysis."

46. Atlas, "Ethics and Access to Teaching Materials."

47. Kevin Coughlin, "Art That Cuts to the Bone: Frank Netter Exhibit at the Morris Museum," Kevco Media LLC, https://morristowngreen.com/2010/11/24/art-that-cuts-to-the-bone-frank-netter-exhibit-at-the-morris-museum/.

48. Ross Eveleth, "Medical Textbooks Overwhelmingly Use Pictures of Young White Men," https://www.vice.com/en_us/article/3k3kkn/medical-textbooks-overwhelmingly-use-pictures-of-young-white-men.

49. Roni C. Rabin, "Dermatology Has a Problem with Skin Color," *New York Times,* Aug. 30, 2020.

50. Stephen B. Thomas and Sandra C. Quinn, "The Tuskegee Syphilis Study, 1932 to 1972: Implications for HIV Education and AIDS Risk Education Programs in the Black Community," *American Journal of Public Health* 81, no. 11 (1991): 1498–505, https://doi.org/10.2105/ajph.81.11.1498.

51. Raymond Evans, "What's with the Blue White Guy in Anatomic Models?," in *Chicago Medical Graphics* (video), ed. Peg Gerrity (Chicago: AMI Diversity: Association of Medical Illustrators, 2021), https://vimeo.com/512297042.

4. The Bright Side of Medical Illustration

1. Max Brödel, "The Intrinsic Blood Vessels of the Kidney and Their Significance in Nephrotomy," *Bulletin of the Johns Hopkins Hospital* 12, no. 118 (1901): 251–60, https://collections.nlm.nih.gov/catalog/nlm:nlmuid-101648447-bk.

2. Edward H. Richardson, "A Simplified Technique for Abdominal Panhysterectomy," *Surgery Gynecology & Obstetrics* 47 (1929): 248–56.

3. Thomas S. Cullen and Max Brödel, "Lesions of the Rectus Abdominis Muscle Simulating an Acute Intra-abdominal Condition. I. Anatomy of the Rectus Muscle," *Bulletin of the Johns Hopkins Hospital* 61, no. 295 (1937): 317–48.

4. Thomas S. Cullen, *Embryology, Anatomy, and Diseases of the Umbilicus: Together with Diseases of the Urachus* (Philadelphia: W. B. Saunders, 1916): ix–x.

5. Patrick C. Walsh, "The Discovery of the Cavernous Nerves and Development of Nerve Sparing Radical Retropubic Prostatectomy," *Journal of Urology* 177, no. 5 (2007): 1632–35, https://doi.org/10.1016/j.juro.2007.01.012.

6. Patrick C. Walsh, "Perfecting Nerve-Sparing Radical Prostatectomy: Sailing in Uncharted Waters," *The Canadian Journal of Urology* 15, no. 5 (2008): 4230–32.

7. Elizabeth M. Ramsey and Ranice W. Crosby, *The Placenta: Human and Animal* (New York: Praeger, 1982).

8. Reuben D. Johnson and Willow Sainsbury, "The 'Combined Eye' of Surgeon and Artist: Evaluation of the Artists Who Illustrated for Cushing, Dandy and Cairns," *Journal of Clinical Neurosciences* 19, no. 1 (2012): 34–38, https://doi.org/10.1016/j.jocn.2011.03.042.

9. Ian Suk, Ziya L. Gokaslan, Gary P. Lees, and Corinne Sandone, "The Art of the Critique: Techniques-Based Tools for Critical Thinking," *Journal of Biocommunication* 36, no. 3 (2010): E81–E94.

10. R. M. Kretzer, Ranice W. Crosby, David A. Rini, and Rafael J. Tamargo, "Dorcas Hager Padget: Neuroembryologist and Neurosurgical Illustrator Trained at Johns Hopkins," *Journal of Neurosurgery* 100, no. 4 (2004): 719–30, https://doi.org/10.3171/jns.2004.100.4.0719.

11. Dorcas H. Padget, "Development of So-Called Dysraphism; with Embryologic Evidence of Clinical Arnold-Chiari and Dandy-Walker Malformations," *Johns Hopkins Medical Journal* 130, no. 3 (1972): 127–65.

12. Karl Grob, Tim Ackland, Markus S. Kuster, Mirjana Manestar, and Luis Filgueira, "A Newly Discovered Muscle: The Tensor of the Vastus Intermedius," *Clinical Anatomy* 29, no. 2 (2016): 256–63, https://doi.org/10.1002/ca.22680.

13. Matthijs H. Valstar, Bernadette S. de Bakker, Roel J. H. M. Steenbakkers, et al., "The Tubarial Salivary Glands: A Potential New Organ at Risk for Radiotherapy," *Radiotherapy and Oncology* 154 (2020): 292–98, https://doi.org/10.1016/j.radonc.2020.09.034.

14. David M. Glover, "The 350th Anniversary of Scientific Publishing: Van Leeuwenhoek, the Most Prolific Author of the Philosophical Transactions of the Royal Society," *Open Biology* 5, no. 4 (2015): 1–2, https://doi.org/10.1098/rsob.150044.

15. Terry S. Yoo, Donald Bliss, Bradley C. Lowekamp, et al., "Visualizing Cells and Humans in 3D: Biomedical Image Analysis at Nanometer and Meter Scales," *IEEE Computer Graphics and Applications* 32, no. 5 (2012): 39–49, https://doi.org/10.1109/MCG.2012.68. Richard L. Felts, Kedar Narayan, Jacob D. Estes, et al., "3D Visualization of HIV Transfer at the Virological Synapse Between Dendritic Cells and T Cells," *Proceedings of the National Academy of Sciences USA* 107, no. 30 (2010): 13336–41, https://doi.org/10.1073/pnas.1003040107.

16. Veronica Falconieri Hays, *How I Built a 3-D Model of the Coronavirus for Scientific American* (New York: Springer Nature America, Inc., 2020).

17. Falconieri Hays, *How I Built a 3-D Model of the Coronavirus*.

18. Martin Kemp, "Kendrew Constructs; Geis Gazes," *Nature* 396, no. 6711 (1998): 525, https://doi.org/10.1038/25019.

19. Makio Murayama, "Molecular Mechanism of Red Cell 'Sickling,'" *Science* 153, no. 3732 (1966): 145–49, https://doi.org/10.1126/science.153.3732.145.

20. Michael Lee and Ashwin Kulshrestha, "Protein Pioneer Jane Richardson Celebrates 50 Years at Duke," *Chronicle*, Nov. 13, 2018.

21. Jane S. Richardson, David C. Richardson, Neil B. Tweedy, et al., "Looking at Proteins: Representations, Folding, Packing, and Design," Biophysical Society National Lecture, *Biophysical Journal* 63, no. 5 (1992): 1185–209, https://pubmed.ncbi.nlm.nih.gov/1477272.

22. James D. Watson and Francis H. Crick, "Molecular Structure of Nucleic Acids: A Structure for Deoxyribose Nucleic Acid," *Nature* 171, no. 4356 (1953): 737–38, https://doi.org/10.1038/171737a0.

23. Kindra Crick, "Quick View: Kindra Crick," *SciArt Initiative,* https://www.sciartmagazine.com/quick-view-kindra-crick.html.

24. David S. Goodsell, Shuchismita Dutta, Christine Zardecki, Maria Voigt, Helen M. Berman, and Stephen K. Burley, "The RCSB PDB 'Molecule of the Month': Inspiring a Molecular View of Biology," *PLoS Biology* 13, no. 5 (2015): e1002140–e1002140, https://doi.org/10.1371/journal.pbi0.1002140.

25. David S. Goodsell, Ludovic Autin, and Arthur J. Olson, "Illustrate: Software for Biomolecular Illustration," *Structure* 27, no. 11 (2019): 1716–20.e1, https://doi.org/10.1016/j.str.2019.08.011.

26. David S. Goodsell, Margaret A. Franzen, and Tim Herman, "From Atoms to Cells: Using Mesoscale Landscapes to Construct Visual Narratives," *Journal of Molecular Biology* 430, no. 21 (2018): 3954–68, https://doi.org/10.1016/j.jmb.2018.06.009.

27. "Beautiful, but Deadly: Painting the Coronavirus," *California Science Weekly,* May 20, 2020.

5. A Universal Language

1. Arianna Selagea, Leah Lebowicz, Samantha Bond, and John Daugherty, "Using Drawing as an Active Engagement Tool to Empower Learners and Promote Teaching of Health Topics," *Journal of Biocommunication* 43, no. 2 (2019): https://doi.org/10.5210/jbc.v43i2.10172.

2. Christoph Niemann, "You Are Fluent in This Language (and Don't Even Know It)," TED, https://www.ted.com/talks/christoph_niemann_you_are_fluent_in_this_language_and_don_t_even_know_it.

3. Gina Roberts-Grey, "Is There Still a Place for the Head Mirror?," *ENT Today: Triological Society,* July 3, 2015.

4. Niemann, "You Are Fluent in This Language."

5. Constantine Mavroudis, Gary P. Lees, and Rachel Idriss, "Medical Illustration in the Era of Cardiac Surgery," *World Journal for Pediatric & Congenital Heart Surgery* 11, no. 2 (2020): 204–14, https://doi.org/10.1177/2150135119893671.

6. Andrew M. Ibrahim and Steven M. Bradley, "Adoption of Visual Abstracts at Circulation CQO: Why and How We're Doing It," *Circulation, Cardiovascular Quality and Outcomes* 10, no. 3 (2017): https://doi.org/10.1161/circoutcomes.117.003684.

7. David Remnick, "David Remnick Looks Back on Tough Decisions as the *New Yorker* Turns 90," Feb. 18, 2015, in *Fresh Air: National Public Radio,* ed. T. Gross, https://www.npr.org/2015/02/18/387229984/david-remnick-looks-back-on-tough-decisions-as-the-new-yorker-turns-90. David Remnick, "95% of *New Yorker* Readers Read the Cartoons First. The Other 5% Are Lying," http://newyorkeronthetown.com/rsvp/kidtooning9/.

8. Ibrahim and Bradley, "Adoption of Visual Abstracts at Circulation CQO."

Valentin Fuster and Douglas Mann, "The Art and Challenge of Crafting a Central Illustration or Visual Abstract," *Journal of the American College of Cardiology* 74, no. 22 (2019): 2816–20, https://doi.org/10.1016/j.jacc.2019.10.035. A. M. Ibrahim, "Visual Abstract," Jan. 2018, https://www.surgeryredesign.com/resources. Lee A. Lindquist and Vanessa Ramirez-Zohfeld, "Visual Abstracts to Disseminate Geriatrics Research through Social Media," *Journal of the American Geriatrics Society* 67, no. 6 (2019): 1128–31, https://doi.org/10.1111/jgs.15853. K Bucher, "Visual Abstracts," presented at SciVizNYC, New York, Nov. 22, 2019.

9. Bucher, "Visual Abstracts." Ibrahim, "Visual Abstract."

10. "Statement on Operating Room Attire," *Bulletin of the American College of Surgeons* 101, no. 10 (2016): 47.

11. Troy A. Markel, Thomas Gormley, Damon Greeley, John Ostojic, Angie Wise, Jonathan Rajala, Rahul Bharadwaj, and Jennifer Wagner, "Hats Off: A Study of Different Operating Room Headgear Assessed by Environmental Quality Indicators," *Journal of the American College of Surgeons* 225, no. 5 (2017): 573–81, https://doi.org/10.1016/j.jamcollsurg.2017.08.014.

12. Robert A. Weber, Stacy Wong, Samantha J. Allen, and Douglas S. Fornfeist," "Assessing the Correlation between a Surgeon's Ability to Draw a Procedure and Ability to Perform the Procedure," *Journal of Surgical Education* 77, no. 3 (2020): 635–42, https://doi.org/10.1016/j.jsurg.2019.12.010.

6. Grammar and Syntax of Medical Illustration

1. Ian Suk, Ziya L. Gokaslan, Gary P. Lees, and Corinne Sandone, "The Art of the Critique: Techniques-Based Tools for Critical Thinking," *The Journal of Biocommunication* 36, no. 3 (2010): E81–E94.

2. François I. Luks, Yvette K. Wild, George J. Piasecki, and Monique E. De Paepe, "Short-Term Tracheal Occlusion Corrects Pulmonary Vascular Anomalies in the Fetal Lamb with Diaphragmatic Hernia," Surgery 128, no. 2 (2000): 266–72, https://doi.org/10.1067/msy.2000.107373.

3. Congenital Diaphragmatic Hernia (CDH), UCSF Benioff Children's Hospitals, https://fetus.ucsf.edu/cdh.

4. François I. Luks and Anthony A. Caldamone, "Undescended Testis," in *Fundamentals of Pediatric Surgery,* 2nd ed., ed. P. Mattei, P. F. Nichol, M. D. I. Rollins, and C. S. Muratore (New York: Springer International Publishing, 2017), 733–39.

5. Left-handed Allen key, April Fool's Day 2012, http://hoaxes.org/af_database/permalink/left_handed_allen_key.

6. Constantine Mavroudis, Gary P. Lees, and Rachid Idriss, "Medical Illustration in the Era of Cardiac Surgery," *World Journal for Pediatric & Congenital Heart Surgery* 11, no. 2 (2020): 204–14, https://doi.org/10.1177/2150135119893671.

7. The Physician as Visual Communicator

1. Josh Ettinger, "What Hollywood Can Teach Researchers about Scientific Storytelling," *Nature,* June 9, 2020, https://doi.org/10.1038/d41586-020-01731-9.

2. Ettinger, "What Hollywood Can Teach Researchers."

3. Jim Harvey, "The Problem for Prezi—Most Prezis Look Rubbish and Don't Work," *PresentationGuru,* May 20, 2016, https://www.presentation-guru.com/the-problem-for-prezi-most-look-rubbish/.

4. Betsy Palay and Tami Tolpa, S. P. A. R. K.: 5 Strategies for the Visual Communication of Science," *Picture as Portal,* https://www.pictureasportal.com/.

5. James L. Boyer, "Bile Formation and Secretion," *Comprehensive Physiology* 3, no. 3 (2013): 1035–78, https://doi.org/10.1002/cphy.c120027.

6. William H. Admirand, "Causes and Management of Gallstones," *Western Journal of Medicine* 124, no. 4 (1976): 330–32.

7. Martin C. Carey, "Pathogenesis of Gallstones," *Recenti Progressi in Medicina* 83, no. 7–8 (1992): 379–91.

8. William H. Admirand and Donald M. Small, "The Physicochemical Basis of Cholesterol Gallstone Formation in Man," *Journal of Clinical Investigation* 47, no. 5 (1968): 1043–52, https://doi.org/10.1172/jci105794.

9. Holly Quinton, "Why I Use Drawing and Creative Processes during the GP Consultation," *British Journal of General Practice* 70, no. 700 (2020): 550, https://doi.org/10.3399/bjgp20X713273.

10. "Zombie Preparedness," Centers for Disease Control and Prevention, https://www.cdc.gov/cpr/zombie/index.htm.

11. Miriam Waite, "Writing Medical Comics," *Journal of Visual Communication in Medicine* 42, no. 3 (2019): 144–50, https://doi.org/10.1080/17453054.2019.1575641.

12. MaryKay Czerwierc, @ComicNurse, https://comicnurse.com/blog/.

13. MaryKay Czerwiec and Michelle N. Huang, "Hospice Comics: Representations of Patient and Family Experience of Illness and Death in Graphic Novels," *Journal of Medical Humanities* 38, no. 2 (2017): 95–113, https://doi.org/10.1007/s10912-014-9303-7.

14. "Medicine AoI," *Annals of Graphic Medicine,* American College of Physicians, https://www.acpjournals.org/topic/web-exclusives/annals-graphic-medicine.

15. Scott McCloud, http://scottmccloud.com/.

16. Frank Deng, "Annals Graphic Medicine—The Palliative Path," *Annals of Internal Medicine* 173, no. 4 (2020): W67–W68, https://doi.org/10.7326/g19-0067.

17. Betsy Palay and Tami Tolpa, "Misconceptions in the Visual Communication of Science II: I Need to Know How to Draw in Order to Make an Effective Picture," *Picture as Portal* blog, Sept. 8, 2020 https://pictureasportal.home.blog/2020/09/08/misconceptions-in-the-visual-communication-of-science-ii-i-need-to-know-how-to-draw-in-order-to-make-an-effective-picture/.

8. The Physician as Illustrator

1. Gianluca Nazzaro and Stefano Veraldi, "Frontal Fibrosing Alopecia—the Fashion of the Renaissance," *JAMA Dermatology* 153, no. 11 (2017): 1105, https://doi.org/10.1001/jamadermat01.2017.3751.

2. Ian Suk, Ziya L. Gokaslan, Gary P. Lees, and Corinne Sandone, "The Art of the Critique: Techniques-Based Tools for Critical Thinking," *The Journal of Biocommunication* 36, no. 3 (2010): E81–E94.

3. Suk et al., "The Art of the Critique."

4. Holly Quinton, "Why I Use Drawing and Creative Processes during the GP consultation," *British Journal of General Practice* 70, no. 700 (2020): 550, https://doi.org/10.3399/bjgp20X713273.

5. Robert A. Weber, Stacy Wong, Samantha J. Allen, and Douglas S. Fornfeist, "Assessing the Correlation between a Surgeon's Ability to Draw a Procedure and Ability to Perform the Procedure," *Journal of Surgical Education* 77, no. 3 (2020): https://doi.org/10.1016/j.jsurg.2019.12.010.

6. Mike Rohde, *The Sketchnote Handbook* (Berkeley, CA: Peachpit Press, 2012).

Index

Page references in italics refer to illustrations.